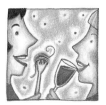

*HEALTH AND HEALING
THE NATURAL WAY*

ENERGIZE
YOUR LIFE

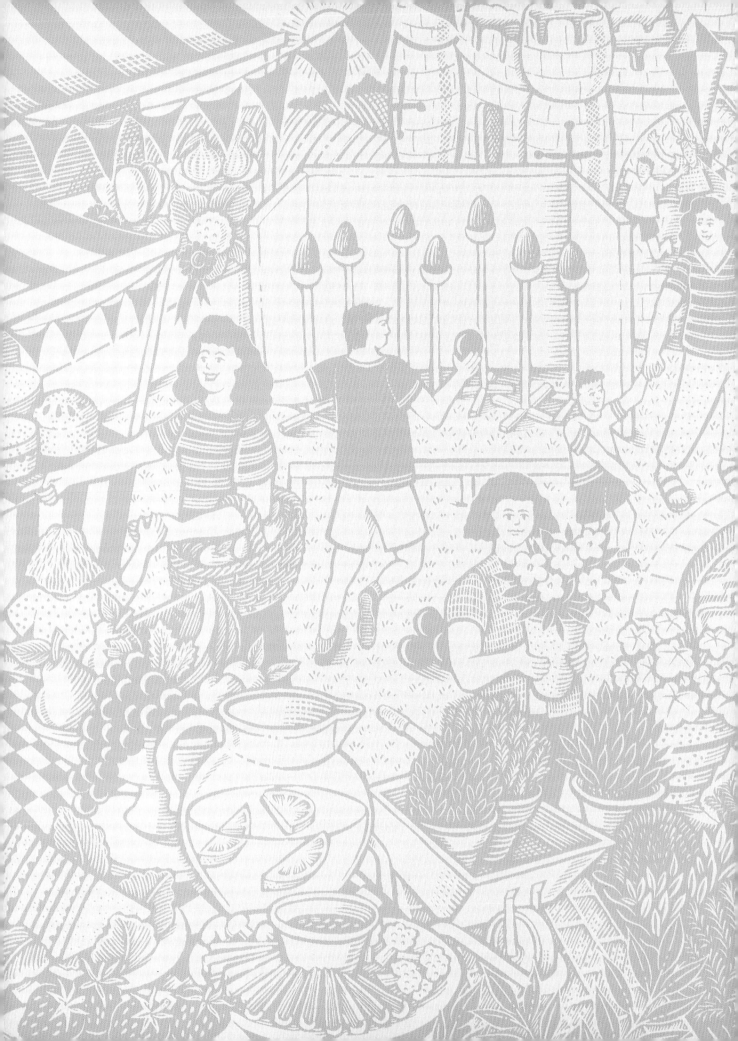

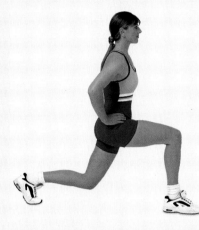

*Health And Healing
The Natural Way*

ENERGIZE
YOUR LIFE

PUBLISHED BY

THE READER'S DIGEST ASSOCIATION, INC.

PLEASANTVILLE, NEW YORK / MONTREAL

A Reader's Digest book
Produced by
Carroll & Brown Limited, London

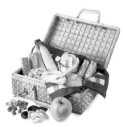

Carroll & Brown

Publishing Director Denis Kennedy
Art Director Chrissie Lloyd

Managing Editor Sandra Rigby
Managing Art Editor Tracy Timson

Editor Jennifer Mussett

Art Editors Mercedes Pearson, Sandra Brooke
Designers Vimit Punater, Julie Bennett

Photographers Jules Selmes, David Murray

Production Wendy Rogers, Clair Reynolds

Computer Management John Clifford,
Paul Stradling, Elisa Merino

The acknowledgments and credits that appear on page 160
are hereby made a part of this copyright page.

Printed in the United States of America
Second Printing, August 2000

Library of Congress Cataloging in Publication Data

Energize your life.
     p.   cm. — (Health and healing the natural way)
Includes index.
ISBN 0-7621-0262-4
  1. Fatigue—Alternative treatment. 2. Naturopathy.
I. Reader's Digest Association.   II. Series.
RB150.F37E54   1999
616' .047—dc21   99-39192

Address any comments about *Energize Your Life* to
Editor in Chief, U.S. Illustrated Reference Books,
Pleasantville, NY 10570.

Consultant

Dr. Michael Jenkins, MBBS, MRCP, FFHom
General practitioner and complementary health specialist

Medical Illustrations Consultant

Dr. Amanda Roberts, MA, MB, BChir

Contributors

Professor Peter O. Behan
MB, ChB, MD, DSc, FRCP (Glas),
FRCP (Lond), FRCP (I)
Professor of Neurology

Dr. Abhijit Chaudhuri
DM, MD, MB, BSc, MRCP (UK)
University lecturer in neurology

Sue Thurgood, BSc, SRD
Senior dietitian

Richard Emerson
Medical health writer

Roger Newman Turner
BAc, ND, DO, MRO, MRN
Registered naturopath, osteopath, and acupuncturist

Reader's Digest Project Staff

Series Editor Gayla Visalli
Editorial Director, health & medicine Wayne Kalyn
Design Director Barbara Rietschel

Reader's Digest Illustrated Reference Books, U.S.

Editor-in-Chief Christopher Cavanagh
Art Director Joan Mazzeo
Operations Manager William J. Cassidy

Reader's Digest Books & Home Entertainment, Canada

Vice President and Editorial Director Deirdre Gilbert
Managing Editor Philomena Rutherford
Art Director John McGuffie

The information in this book is for reference only; it is
not intended as a substitute for a doctor's diagnosis and care.
The editors urge anyone with continuing medical problems
or symptoms to consult a doctor.

ENERGIZE YOUR LIFE

More and more people today are choosing to take greater responsibility for their own health care rather than relying on a doctor to step in with a cure when something goes wrong. We now recognize that we can influence our health by making improvements in lifestyle, such as a better diet, more exercise, and reduced stress. People are also becoming increasingly aware that there are other healing methods—some of them new, others ancient—that can help prevent illness or be used as a complement to orthodox medicine.

The series *Health and Healing the Natural Way* will help you make your own health choices by giving you clear, comprehensive, straightforward, and encouraging infor-mation and advice about methods for improving your health. The series explains the many different natural therapies now available, including aromatherapy, herbalism, acu-pressure, and a number of others, and the circumstances in which they may be of benefit when used in conjunction with conventional medicine.

ENERGIZE YOUR LIFE investigates the causes of and treatments for fatigue and other energy problems and provides suggestions for boosting energy in cases ranging from people who feel tired occasionally to those with a major debilitating condition. All of the main causes of fatigue are covered, including sleeping problems, emotional stress, lifestyle, and illness. There is an in-depth analysis of dietary needs and the use of nutrient supplements in the treatment of energy problems. The book also describes energizing exercises for your body and mind and gives suggestions for reducing stress and other energy drainers in your life. The last chapter of this volume covers medical conditions that can lead to fatigue and some of the alternative therapies that can help alleviate them. *ENERGIZE YOUR LIFE* explains how we can all develop and maintain a more positive outlook to promote improved health and vitality and a sense of balance in life.

CONTENTS

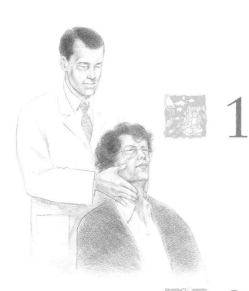

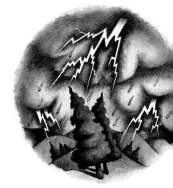

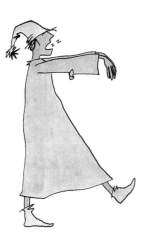

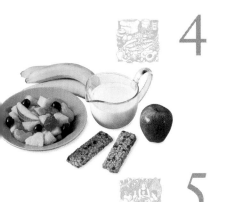

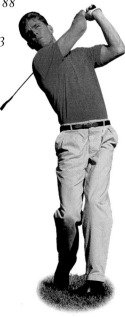

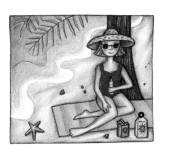

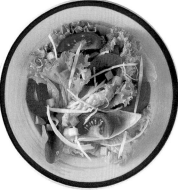

BOOSTING ENERGY LEVELS

Most people would like more energy to cope with life's demands. It is possible to achieve new energy levels, often with just simple changes in lifestyle.

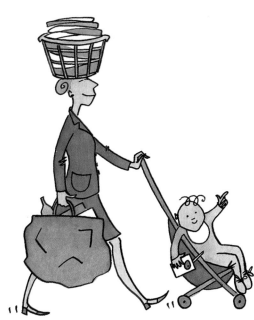

BUSY, BUSY WORLD
More is expected of everyone in today's fast-moving world. Getting everything done and staying on top of commitments can demand high levels of energy.

In recent years lack of energy has become a major health issue. It is one of the most common complaints presented to doctors and is the frequent subject of magazine articles, television talk shows, and self-help books. People often complain that if only they had more energy they could achieve more, be happier, or simply stay on top of existing commitments. Although we all suffer periods of low energy from time to time, for some people loss of energy takes an extreme and disabling form: chronic fatigue syndrome (CFS), also known as myalgic encephalomyelitis (ME).

The existence of chronic fatigue syndrome remains controversial in the eyes of some doctors. Increasingly, however, they are recognizing it as a distinct and diagnosable illness. It is now generally defined as extreme fatigue; in some cases the sufferer is unable even to move without assistance. Exactly what causes CFS is unclear, although it often follows a flulike virus. A number of risk factors have been identified, among them, protracted physical or mental stress, nutritional deficiencies, and allergies. All these things can affect the immune system, and they may make some people vulnerable to extreme fatigue. The condition seems to be on the rise; it is conservatively estimated to affect 40 people out of every 100,000, although U.S. studies suggest that the figure could be as high as 100 per 100,000. In Canada it affects 20,000 to 30,000 adults.

There are many theories about why fatigue is on the increase. Some people believe our modern lifestyle is simply too demanding, that the pace of life causes excessive mental and physical stress, which depletes the immune system. Other people believe that low energy reflects a depressed outlook or poor eating habits or too little or even too much exercise. The reality seems to be that low energy is the result of a complex interaction of all of these factors, and treatments need to encompass the whole person. However, not only are the causes of low energy diverse, but the concept of what we actually mean by "energy" has also broadened. What scientists have learned has had huge implications for the way we look at the world, as well as how we understand our own health and energy levels.

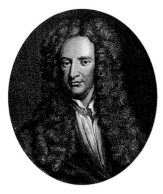

SIR ISAAC NEWTON
One of the greatest scientists in history, Newton believed that everything in the universe was made from solid particles of matter, or atoms.

SIR ISAAC NEWTON AND ENERGY

Until the mid 19th century, our understanding of what energy consisted of and how the physical world worked, even how the human body worked, was reasonably straightforward. The prevailing view of the world was largely based on the work of Sir Isaac Newton. He determined that the world consisted of solid units of matter (atoms); these always remained identical in shape and mass and were acted upon by the force of gravity, which he saw as the essential energy force in the world. He believed that the world ran according to fixed rules, like a giant machine, and that for every observable effect there was an identifiable cause. However, this theory failed to explain powerful energy forces discovered in the 19th century—electric and magnetic phenomena. By the mid-19th century, scientists had realized that the physical world and our own place in it was more complex than they had previously thought.

THE NEW PHYSICS

A radical shift in how science viewed the physical world occurred at the beginning of the 20th century, when Albert Einstein published his theory of relativity and quantum theory. Until Einstein's discoveries, scientists from the time of the ancient Greeks onward believed that all matter was composed of solid particles. Einstein's theories and the work of the physicists who followed him showed that, far from being solid, atoms consist of vast regions of space in which extremely small particles called electrons move around the atom's nucleus. Further research revealed that fundamentally it is energy—the force of electrical attraction between the nucleus of each atom and the electrons traveling around it—that forms the basis not only of all solids, liquids, and gases but also of all living things and the biological processes that bring them into existence.

ALBERT EINSTEIN
Revolutionizing modern thinking, Einstein discovered that every particle of matter is charged with electromagnetic energy.

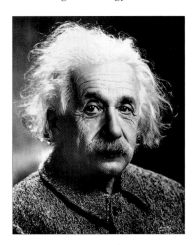

Human beings are essentially composed of and subject to the same basic energy forces as all animate and inanimate matter, and the entire universe is united by the principal force of energy.

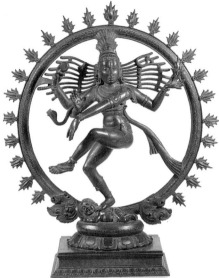

SHIVA
This statuette depicts Shiva, the Hindu god symbolizing the unity of opposites.

Einstein's theory of relativity demonstrated that this energy was constantly dynamic, constantly changing matter into different forms and states.

PARALLELS WITH EASTERN RELIGIONS

In reaching this radical new understanding of the world, the new physics has been observed to have many parallels with astern thought and religion. In 1974 physicist Fritjof Capra was first to explore these parallels in his best-selling book, *The Tao hysics*. He argued that religions such as Buddhism, Hinduism, Taoism all place dynamic energy at the center of the universe, see all things—food, the seasons, people, even the arrangement of furniture in our houses—as being imbued with and subject to dynamic, constantly changing energy, and that this was just one of many similarities between modern physics and ancient religions.

The complexity of modern physics is daunting, yet the more we learn about what affects our own energy levels, the more these theories seem to make sense. Our fluctuating energy levels cannot be explained by any one factor: all the forces and elements we interact with—the people we meet, the emotions we experience, the seasons, and the food we eat—influence our level of energy. The holistic way of looking at health is embodied in Ayurvedic medicine and traditional Chinese medicine.

HEALTHY DIET
Energy comes from the food we eat. The better the quality of fuel we consume, in the form of fresh fruits and vegetables and grains, the higher our energy levels.

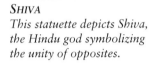

THE HUMAN BODY AND ENERGY

Your energy relates directly to the amount and type of food you eat. This link has always been apparent to even the most primitive societies, although exactly how food was digested and energy gained was not understood. The ancient Greeks were the first to experiment with digestion, and the physician Galen calculated digestion rates in the stomach but wrongly believed that the nourishment from food was absorbed, transformed into a milky liquid, and passed into the liver, where it was imbued with a natural spirit that produced energy. The Renaissance brought a new wave of medical research, and Italian academics proposed that the digestive system worked like a machine, although the soul was still named as the driving force behind it. It was not until the early 19th century that the

American surgeon William Beaumont made headway into understanding the digestive processes. His research formed the basis for the work of the French scientist Claude Bernard, who made the breakthrough discovery that all food is absorbed into the blood and taken to the liver, where it is transformed into sugar and glycogen, which can be used to form energy.

The vital role that oxygen plays in food digestion was first discovered in the 18th century by the Irish scientist Robert Boyle. Then early in the 19th century, the Italian physicist and priest Lazzaro Spallanzani reached the conclusion that the transformation of food into energy takes place in every tissue in the body as oxygen is transformed into carbon dioxide.

The exact process by which each cell produces energy was not discovered until after the Second World War, when powerful microscopes and research instruments allowed scientists to observe the action of cells for the first time. The role of hormones (the name is derived from the Greek word meaning "to excite") in controlling metabolism and energy production was first identified in the 18th century, but the individual hormones and their functions were not established until the 20th century.

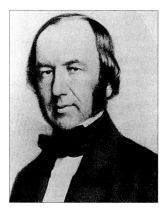

CLAUDE BERNARD
The great physiologist Claude Bernard made important advances in the fields of digestion and energy, hormones and metabolism.

THE HUMAN MIND AND ENERGY

Our understanding of how the mind affects energy has developed more slowly. The ancient Greeks recognized the importance of the brain as the center of intellectual life and the seat of the soul. Some philosophers thought that sleep occurred because of a temporary retreat of blood from the brain and that death indicated a permanent departure. Diseases of the brain, such as epilepsy, were known as "sacred" diseases, and the actions associated with them were believed to spring from the brain. The physician Galen described an "animal spirit" in the brain that was concerned with intellectual activities, sensation, and movement.

During the Renaissance and Enlightenment, philosophers further analyzed brain functioning and how the brain interacts with the nervous system and metabolism. However, the human psyche and thought processes—how we feel, think, and make decisions— were not fully investigated until the early 20th century,

PSYCHOTHERAPY
Research has proved that positive emotional experiences and an optimistic mental attitude can dramatically improve energy levels.

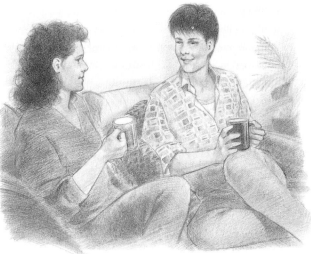

when Sigmund Freud dared to analyze the human mind. The conclusion of Freud's research—namely, that each person reacts to situations according to his or her own personal experiences and physical and emotional needs—led to a surge in psychiatric and neurochemical analysis. It is now known that the mind plays an enormous role in the health and energy of the individual, through hormone secretions in the brain, as well as thoughts and feelings, and the influence that these have on the body. Further research is needed to understand these processes more fully. It is now clear, however, that patients with low energy levels often benefit from psychotherapy or stress relief to help them deal with their problems and address any hidden emotional agenda.

CREATING A HIGH-ENERGY LIFESTYLE

Whether you are suffering from sporadic tiredness or experiencing a general and prolonged lack of energy, you can make a number of simple adjustments to your lifestyle that may dramatically improve your vitality. ENERGIZE YOUR LIFE will help you to identify what changes would be most appropriate for maximizing your energy levels. Every aspect of how and where energy is required, produced, and used in the body is covered in detail, making it possible to understand how you can better maintain your vim and vigor.

Chapter 1 looks at how energy is produced. Every person has different energy levels and food needs, depending on his or her energy expenditure. Your hormonal status, including your sexual hormones, play a large part in energy balance, and understanding your body can help you to adapt to hormonal changes, such as those that accompany menstruation or old age.

Chapter 2 investigates natural energy sources and how they have been used in certain cultures and for energy therapies. Chapter 3 covers potential energy drainers in your life, such as sleeping problems, caffeine, and emotional disruption.

Chapter 4 considers healthy nutrition, focusing on the nutrients that you need for energy and how to prevent debilitating deficiencies. Exercises for physical and mental energy, including relaxation techniques, are covered in Chapter 5. Chapter 6 describes the more serious conditions that are associated with low energy, such as chronic fatigue syndrome and anemia, and what you can do about them.

POSITIVE RELATIONSHIPS
Sharing positive energies with others and avoiding negative feelings can help you stay happy and energized.

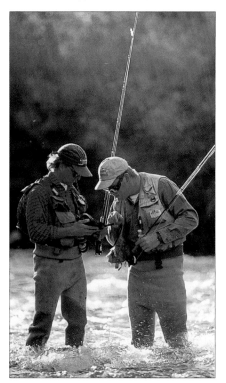

ARE YOU MAKING THE MOST OF YOUR ENERGY POTENTIAL?

How often do you feel tired and unable to do the things that you usually enjoy? Most people experience a period of low energy occasionally, but for some the condition is chronic. There is much you can do to maintain your zest. Understanding how you gain and expend energy can help you to acquire good health and vitality, allowing you to pursue and achieve your goals.

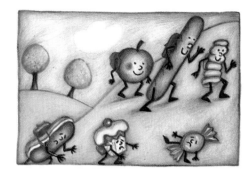

Q ARE YOU GETTING THE RIGHT QUANTITIES AND TYPES OF FOOD?

Your primary source of energy is the food that you eat, but much depends on how well it is digested. For maximum energy potential, the best foods are complex carbohydrates, such as bread, pasta, and rice, and plenty of fruits, vegetables, nuts, and beans. Refined sugar and foods that are high in it, such as cake and candy, offer nothing but a sugar rush, which can leave you feeling even more tired and low in blood sugar a few hours later. A healthy balanced diet is the best grounding for high energy levels (see Chapter 4).

Q ARE YOU GETTING ENOUGH NUTRIENTS?

Nutrients play a crucial role in the functioning of everyday bodily processes, including food absorption, energy production, and proper mental functioning. If your energy levels are low, you may not be getting all the minerals and vitamins that you need in your diet. You can rectify this by adjusting your diet to include foods rich in nutrients or by taking supplements if necessary. You may also suffer from mild nutrient deficiencies if your body is not absorbing the nutrients from food properly. This may be caused by other nutritional deficiencies, excessive alcohol intake, smoking, or an undetected medical condition. Chapter 4 details the essential nutrients for health and energy.

Q DO YOU FEEL OUT OF BREATH IF YOU RUN UP SOME STAIRS?

Your body becomes more energized the more it is used, so it pays to build more exercise into your routine (see Chapter 5). Doing exercise regularly and raising your heartbeat for more than 20 minutes three times a week will give you the vitality that you need for your everyday life.

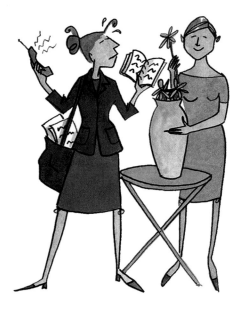

Q DO YOU WASTE ENERGY DOING THINGS THAT YOU DON'T HAVE TO DO?

You may be wasting energy on things that are not significant in your life. Worrying about unimportant issues, getting upset or distracted by others, and feeling guilty about your own actions are all negative aspects that can drain your energy before you get a chance to do the things that are important to you. Sorting the negative from the positive feelings and not allowing unnecessary worries to drain you physically can help you find more energy. Motivating yourself with new challenges or rewarding yourself when you meet your own personal goals can work miracles in finding new reserves of untapped energy. Taking up new pastimes or hobbies or perhaps even changing jobs can help you to channel your energy and challenge yourself with new experiences.

Q DO YOU THINK YOU MAY HAVE A MORE SERIOUS MEDICAL PROBLEM?

Fatigue is a symptom of many medical conditions, a sign that the body is attempting to counteract the effects of an illness, disease, or deficiency. Locating and treating the cause of fatigue can be difficult, although many tests are available for diagnosing specific conditions so that they can be properly treated. Several of the physical problems associated with fatigue are discussed in Chapter 6, which also examines chronic fatigue syndrome. For many conditions, dietary changes, herbal supplements, and other complementary therapies can do a great deal to relieve symptoms, although you should always consult your doctor first if you are suffering from fatigue for no apparent reason.

Q DO YOU GET ENOUGH REST AND RELAXATION?

When you are tired, do you rest properly or merely sit down and worry about your problems? Proper rest and relaxation means resting your body, your mind, and your emotions—giving yourself a complete break from life's ups and downs. This can be achieved by mental relaxation exercises, such as meditation, yoga, and chi kung (see Chapter 5), which aim to raise you above day-to-day worries. A good night's sleep without the use of pills is fundamental, and if you have trouble sleeping or wake up often, you might consider the action steps described in Chapter 3. Sleep is one of the first things that people skip if they have a busy schedule, although they rarely consider the broader effects that lack of sleep has on their lives and energy levels.

CHAPTER 1

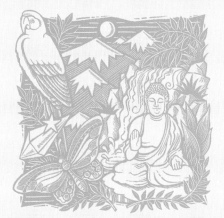

ENERGY AND THE INDIVIDUAL

Every process and movement of the body—the ability to think, feel, work, and play—is fueled by energy that comes from food and beverages. Certain cells break down and convert food into a form that can be used for living. But other factors, both internal and external, also affect the amount of energy you have at different stages of your life.

WHAT IS ENERGY?

Energy makes all activity possible; anything that moves or grows uses energy to do so. When energy is at a peak, not only will you feel vital, but your general health will be excellent.

Energy forms the basis of our lives. All life on earth is based on systems of energy that provide light and warmth and enable growth, movement, and action. Energy is needed for lighting and heating our homes and workplaces, transporting us, and growing and processing food to nourish us. Energy is also the basis of the body's own systems: it keeps us alive and functioning efficiently and effectively.

Ultimately all energy on earth, including the energy that sustains our bodies, derives either directly or indirectly from the sun. For example, fuels such as coal and oil were formed millions of years ago from vegetation. When oil or coal is burned as fuel, the energy released is derived from the sun's rays that were absorbed by prehistoric trees and plants. In the same way, much of our own energy supply is derived from the sun's energy absorbed by the plants we eat today. Plants use the light from the sun to make sugars from carbon dioxide and water.

THE LAWS OF ENERGY

Because energy is so all-encompassing in our lives, it is difficult to define precisely. However, scientists have determined a number of laws about how energy works. These laws can be applied to understanding how energy works in our own bodies.

First, energy cannot be created from nothing. Things do not become energized by themselves but are acted upon by other forces. For example, a toy car cannot start to move by itself: either it is propelled by an internal slow-release spring or a battery that utilizes chemical energy, or it is moved by a child using his or her own energy to push or pull it. Although this process may seem obvious, it is a point many people forget when they are under pressure from work or family commitments. If they eat poorly or irregularly and get inadequate rest, they are asking their body to create energy from nothing and will end up tired and run-down.

If energy cannot be created from nothing, where does it come from? The answer is—another energy source. The second law of energy is that it can be changed from one form to another. For example, winding up (applying mechanical energy to) a spring in a clockwork car creates potential kinetic energy (the energy of moving objects); the car now holds the future ability to move. Once the spring is released and the car is moving, it has kinetic energy, which was derived from mechanical energy.

Another example of energy conversion is the process of photosynthesis, whereby molecules in plants chemically convert the light energy from the sun into sugars, which in turn can be converted in the body to other types of energy. Some sugars may be transformed into heat energy to maintain our body at the correct temperature; others may become kinetic energy when we take a walk; and some may be stored in our cells, to be released as our body requires more energy.

The third energy principle is that of conservation. Expressed simply, this means that although energy can be changed into different forms, the amount of energy after the change is equal to the amount of energy at the start. So if we eat foods of low caloric value or ones that our bodies find difficult to convert, we will be able to produce only a low level of energy and will lack vitality.

Of course, the human body is far more complex than a plant. Its energy levels are also affected by the intricate workings of the brain. Many people underestimate the draining effects of prolonged emotional stress, for example. Your body responds to stress with the physical reactions of

FEELING ENERGY
Your energy levels are the result of many factors: the air that you breathe, the food that you eat, as well as your emotional state.

increased heart and breathing rates and raised blood pressure. Your liver also releases energy-giving sugars to boost your general energy levels. This response causes a huge drain in your energy supplies. Even though emotions may seem quite separate from physical processes, in fact they have a very real impact on bodily health, especially on hormone secretion and energy.

We are also affected by external energy forces, in addition to the food we eat. For instance, medical doctors utilize forms of energy to treat some illnesses and diseases. One example is radiation therapy, which makes use of electromagnetic energy to destroy cancerous cells in the body. Many alternative therapists believe, however, that we are influenced by energy in a more integral way. Some see individuals as having their own energy fields and believe that these fields are interacting on a constant basis with all the energy forces of nature. In many Eastern cultures, a pervasive view is that a change in energy levels can occur in relation to seasons and that people should adjust their lifestyle and behavior to correspond with these external changes.

Perhaps the crucial point to remember when thinking about your energy level is that energy is all-encompassing. Energy is influenced by many forces, both external and internal, and the key to good health lies in finding a harmonious balance in these forces that influence our lives.

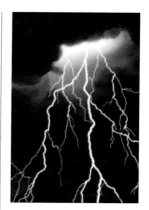

LIGHTNING
Energy is released from highly charged particles in the atmosphere.

FACTORS THAT AFFECT ENERGY

Taking time to organize your life can help you manage your energy better and control factors around you that are affecting your energy levels. Confusion, stress, and not knowing what you want are the greatest of all drains on your energy. Take steps toward conquering them by making a list of the things that you like and want to see happening in your future. If you recognize the factors that affect your energy, you can work out ways to counter them and help to realize your best potential energy levels.

Sleep and rest
It is essential to rest properly in order to restore your body. During sleep your body and mind have time to relax and unwind from stress you may not even be aware that you have experienced.

The seasons
Climate and weather can influence your energy levels. The lack of sunshine in the winter can leave you feeling tired and in need of extra energy boosts during this season.

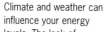

Relationships
Positive relations with those around you can help you feel happy, and a relationship with someone special can add extra zest to your life.

Exercise
Regular exercise, raising your heartbeat for at least 20 minutes three times a week, improves energy levels.

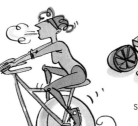

A healthy diet
Providing your body with both sufficient calories and the nutrients that you need for proper functioning are crucial factors for sustaining high energy and health.

Weight watching
Keeping your weight at a normal level for your height and build helps boost your health and energy. Carrying around more weight than you need slows you down and tires you out.

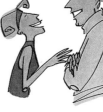

Environmental factors
Living in a healthy environment and setting aside time to enjoy the countryside and natural beauty of the world around you can increase your energy.

Sex
A fulfilling and happy sex life is an important part of personal and emotional health. It can also be fun and relaxing and help you to reaffirm a good relationship.

Fulfilling your potential
Recognizing, pursuing, and ultimately fulfilling your ambitions and dreams can be the most difficult but rewarding challenges of your life. In order to live a balanced, happy, and energized existence, you must realize your potential and reach goals you have set for yourself.

Light and color
Light is an essential element in supplying energy, not just for people but for nearly all life on the planet. Living with colors that help you to feel energized can boost your vitality.

ENERGY AND YOUR BODY

Understanding the processes by which your body gains and expends energy will help you to recognize the factors that cause people to have different energy levels.

The energy that powers your muscles and fuels your brain comes from what you eat. The process begins in your digestive system, where the energy-giving nutrients are extracted from food and passed into your bloodstream. This complex procedure occurs at different rates throughout the day according to your age, state of health, and dietary needs, as well as the type of food that you are eating.

THE DIGESTIVE SYSTEM

The digestive tract, also known as the alimentary canal, consists of a continuous series of tubes, including the stomach, that extend through the body from the mouth to the anus. In adults this tract is more than 10 meters (33 feet) long, and each section of it has a different function.

Other important parts of the digestive system include the teeth, tongue, and salivary glands; the swallowing mechanism in the esophagus (gullet); and the liver and pancreas, which are situated in the abdomen. Digestion begins when you chew your food. Saliva in the mouth starts the chemical breakdown of food with an enzyme (a protein that speeds up chemical reactions) that converts starches to sugars.

When you swallow food, a series of muscular contractions pushes it down your esophagus, the tube that connects the throat to the stomach. Once in your stomach, food is mixed with digestive juices that begin to break it down into its component nutrients. This process is aided by rhythmic movements of the stomach wall.

Some components of food—such as glucose and water—are absorbed directly through the stomach wall and pass into the bloodstream for immediate use by your body, but most of them pass from your stomach into your small intestine. Digestion is completed there with the aid of digestive juices from the liver and pancreas, and the nutrients from food are absorbed into your bloodstream through the intestine wall.

By the time food leaves the small intestine and enters the large intestine (colon), almost all of its usable nutrients have been removed. As food passes through the large intestine, bacteria living there decompose it,

THE DIGESTIVE SYSTEM

Food is absorbed through the digestive system in a variety of ways, usually with the help of enzymes released by the body to aid in the breakdown of food. The food is eventually broken down into glucose, which can be converted into energy with the help of oxygen.

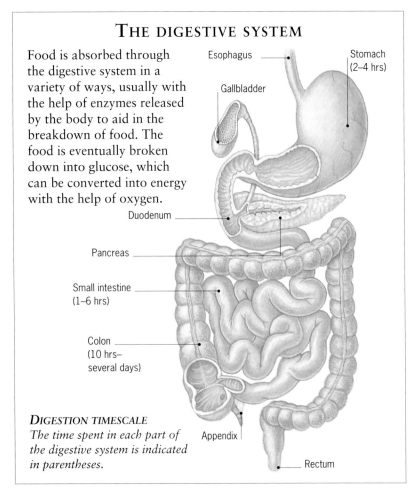

Esophagus

Stomach (2–4 hrs)

Gallbladder

Duodenum

Pancreas

Small intestine (1–6 hrs)

Colon (10 hrs– several days)

Appendix

Rectum

DIGESTION TIMESCALE
The time spent in each part of the digestive system is indicated in parentheses.

a process that produces gas and a few of the B vitamins. By the time the residue of the digested food is expelled from the body, it consists of about 75 percent water and 25 percent solids; the solids are composed mainly of undigested fiber, dead bacteria, fat, some inorganic matter, and a small amount of protein.

BREAKING DOWN FOOD FOR ENERGY

The main sources of energy in food are carbohydrates (sugars and starches) and fats, but some energy also comes from proteins. Carbohydrates, found in such foods as bread, pasta, fruit, potatoes, rice, and beans, are composed of carbon, hydrogen, and oxygen. The most basic forms of carbohydrate are the simple sugars, called monosaccharides. These sugars, which include glucose, are the building blocks of the other carbohydrates. There are also disaccharides—more complex sugars consisting of pairs of monosaccharides—and polysaccharides, or starches, which are made up of long chains of disaccharides.

Fats, from foods such as dairy products, vegetable oils, fish, and meat, are also made up of carbon, hydrogen, and oxygen, but these are combined in more complex ways than in carbohydrates. The basic components of fat are glycerol and fatty acids. Proteins—contained especially in meat, poultry, fish, legumes, and dairy products—are even more complex, being built up from chains of amino acids, which consist of carbon, hydrogen, oxygen, and nitrogen.

In the digestive system, all carbohydrates are broken down into glucose, which passes into the bloodstream (as blood sugar) to be carried around the body as the principal energy source. Fats are broken down into glycerol and fatty acids, and proteins into amino acids. These last are used for maintaining and repairing body tissue, as well as for providing energy.

ENERGY TRANSFER

The energy that powers body cells is a chemical form, released when a substance called adenosine triphosphate (ATP) is

---

DID YOU KNOW?

When Henry VIII died at age 55, he was grossly overweight, thanks to abundant court feasts. As a result, he suffered from kidney disease, gout, circulatory disorders, and a "tortuously painful" leg ulcer, which afflicted him throughout his later years.

Energy and activity
The more active you are, the harder your metabolism has to work to produce the energy you need. On average, a man burns about 90 calories an hour while sitting, 120 standing, 220 walking, and 600 while running. Typically, a woman burns 70 calories an hour while sitting, 100 standing, 180 walking, and 420 running.

AEROBIC AND ANAEROBIC ENERGY

During normal muscle use, including moderate exercise, the series of chemical reactions that convert food into energy for your muscles is an aerobic process; that is, it uses oxygen. The word *aerobic* comes from the Greek word for air. But when you exercise strenuously, your muscles use up oxygen (and glucose) faster than your bloodstream can supply it. When this happens, your muscles run out of energy and rapidly tire. This shortage of energy can be overcome by the action of a backup chemical in the muscles—phosphorylcreatine. This chemical can supply energy when oxygen is in short supply, although only for a short period, such as a sprint. Because this type of energy production requires no oxygen, it is called *anaerobic*.

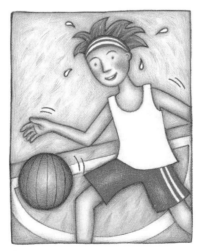

ANAEROBIC EXERCISE
Anaerobic exercise occurs when you exert yourself strenuously for a short period, such as during a sprint down a basketball court or a brief run for a bus.

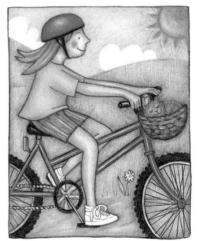

AEROBIC EXERCISE
Bicycle riding, brisk walking, and jogging are all good examples of exercise that uses oxygen, exerting your lungs and heart and improving all-round fitness and health.

OBESITY AND ENERGY LEVELS

Obese people are especially prone to fatigue because the extra pounds they carry make it difficult for them to move easily and they tend to be become less active. As their activity declines, so does their physical fitness; eventually, even minimal exertion can bring on shortness of breath and exhaustion. Besides being easily fatigued, obese people are at greater risk for many disorders, including high blood pressure, heart disease, adult-onset diabetes, gallbladder problems, certain types of cancer, arthritis, and foot and back pain.

ENERGY REQUIREMENTS
People need to consume just enough food to keep their energy supply in line with their expenditure. An active person requires more food, while a sedentary person would quickly become fat on the same diet.

broken down into a simpler substance, adenosine diphosphate (ADP). To keep this energy-producing process going, the ADP is converted back into ATP by the energy released when glucose is broken down and combined with oxygen in the bloodstream. This process allows energy to be steadily released for movement.

As well as delivering oxygen, blood collects carbon dioxide and water—the by-products of the energy-producing process. These are taken away by red blood cells and plasma, the liquid part of the blood that carries the blood cells. This process is therefore dependent on the proper functioning of the blood, particularly the red blood cells, oxygen from the lungs, and glucose and fatty acids from food.

STORING ENERGY

Not all of the energy in the food you eat is required immediately, so your body needs some way of storing the surplus for later use. Surplus glucose, derived from carbohydrates, is converted into glycogen (a complex carbohydrate), which is stored in your muscles and liver. As the glucose in your bloodstream is used up to provide energy, glycogen is converted back into glucose and released into the bloodstream. Glycogen can also be made from protein, after it is first converted into amino acids and glucose, and also from the glycerol in fats.

When glycogen stores are full, any surplus glucose and other energy-producing nutrients are stored as body fat. This fat can then be broken down into glycerol and fatty acids again when it is needed to provide energy.

Body fat takes two forms, brown and white, and is stored in layers of cells under the skin, especially on the buttocks and around the kidneys and heart. Brown fat, a kind of medium-term energy reserve, is the first to be used when blood glucose levels are running low, for instance, when you have been exercising hard or have not eaten for some time. White fat, the type that causes

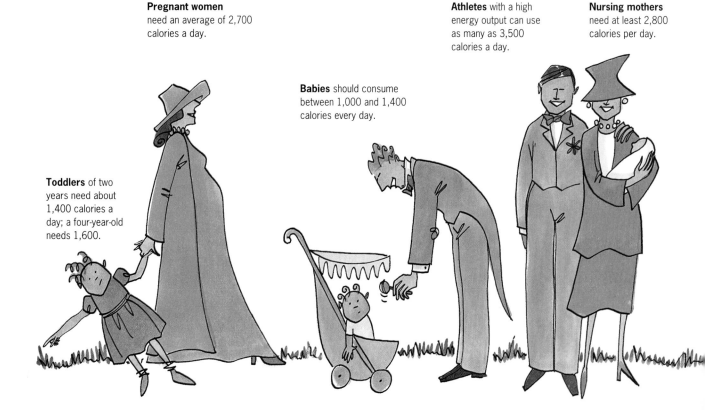

Pregnant women need an average of 2,700 calories a day.

Babies should consume between 1,000 and 1,400 calories every day.

Athletes with a high energy output can use as many as 3,500 calories a day.

Nursing mothers need at least 2,800 calories per day.

Toddlers of two years need about 1,400 calories a day; a four-year-old needs 1,600.

obesity, is a long-term store. Your body builds up this type of energy reserve when the brown fat cells are full.

A healthy level of body fat is good because it protects the body against cold and physical harm and acts as a reserve store of energy. However, many people have a tendency to store too much fat, and this condition leads to the health problems associated with being overweight.

METABOLISM

Metabolism consists of catabolic and anabolic processes. Catabolism takes place when energy is produced by the breaking down of complex substances into simpler ones, such as the conversion of glucose into carbon dioxide and water. In contrast, anabolism is the use of energy to build up simple substances into more complex ones—for example, when amino acids, which are produced from food proteins by catabolism, are reassembled into body-building proteins for making muscle tissue.

The amount of energy your metabolism produces over a given time is known as your metabolic rate. When you are resting, your metabolism is producing just the energy needed to sustain vital functions such as breathing, heartbeat, digestion, and maintenance of body temperature. The amount of energy you produce and use when you are resting is your basal metabolic rate (BMR), which varies according to age, height, weight, sex, and such factors as pregnancy and breast-feeding a baby.

As soon as you start to move about, your metabolic rate increases to provide the extra energy you need. This increase is triggered by the action of hormones such as adrenaline, insulin, steroids, and thyroxine.

When your metabolic rate rises, your body responds by converting food or fat reserves into energy. If your intake and output of energy are about equal, then you will have a healthy weight. If you eat less than you need for energy, you will lose weight. This is the basis of the concept of a calorie-controlled diet. If, on the other hand, you are eating more than you burn up, the excess energy will be stored as fat on your body. This happens often with people as they get older and become less active but do not reduce the amount of food they eat.

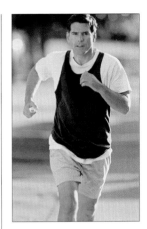

KEEPING ACTIVE
Exercising aerobically for at least 20 to 30 minutes three times a week will improve your body's ability to produce energy.

DID YOU KNOW?

The 400-meter race is known to be one of the most difficult because it is too long to run anaerobically and yet too short to be an aerobic exercise. Most runners use a combination of aerobic and anaerobic energy to cover the distance. When to begin the final sprint is considered a tactical and crucial point for success.

Children between the ages of 7 and 10 need 1,600 to 2,400 calories per day.

Teenagers between 14 and 18 need 2,200 calories a day if female and 2,700 a day if male.

An adult woman needs an average of 2,100 calories a day.

An adult man needs an average of 2,800 calories per day.

Middle-aged people over 50 years old need about 1,800 calories if female and 2,500 if male.

Elderly people over age 70 need only 1,500 calories a day for a man, 1,200 for a woman.

GROWING NEEDS

Children require large amounts of calories and protein relative to their weight and height to enable them to grow and be active. As girls enter puberty, their protein needs level off and their caloric requirements decline. Boys usually require more food than girls during puberty in order to develop and maintain more muscle mass, and these needs don't taper off until boys enter early adulthood.

CALORIE INTAKE
Calories are the energy-producing elements in your diet. They will be stored as fat if they are not used.

PROTEIN NEEDS
Protein is needed not only for growth but also for proper functioning of the body and for repairing tissues. It can also be used as a source of energy.

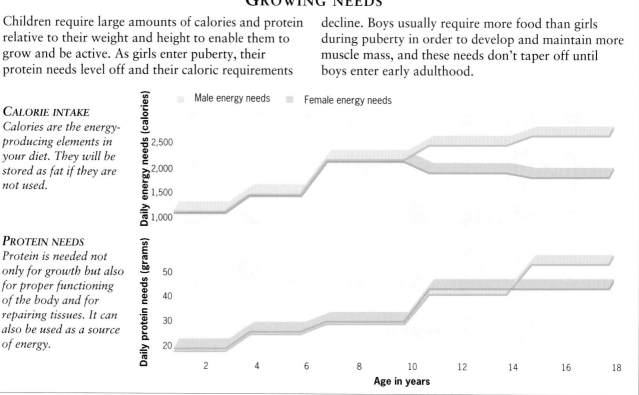

ENERGY REQUIREMENTS AND AGE

Children have a higher BMR than grownups, and their diets should include slightly more fat and sugar than an adult's diet. Children entering puberty and in their early teens have a lower BMR than younger ones, but their need for calcium remains high because the bones are still growing. A diet high in all nutrients is needed during the growth spurt at puberty. Teenage girls in particular require large amounts of minerals and vitamins (but not necessarily calories), especially iron, magnesium, and the B vitamins, to help their bodies cope with the onset of menstruation. Boys, on the other hand, have rapidly growing muscle mass and height during this time, and their calorie as well as nutritional demands can be huge.

The BMR declines after puberty and in most people continues to decline gradually until middle age, when energy requirements begin to decrease more rapidly. Past age 50, everyone experiences a reduction in body tissue, particularly muscle mass and bone density, and a decrease in the efficiency of the organs. More fat develops, and there is a trend toward changes in the hormone levels affecting all glands, particularly the thyroid (see page 140). This is a gradual process, and its rate of progression varies widely; some individuals appear to be healthier and less affected by these changes than others.

Modern research has shown that there is no single factor that brings about the cellular changes of aging, although a poor diet, environmental factors, and lack of exercise can all have an effect.

ENERGY BOOST

Visit a swimming pool for exercise. Water provides a supportive environment for muscles and joints, allowing you to move without putting strain on any part of your body. It can be particularly beneficial if you have arthritis or are recovering from an injury and cannot exercise in the normal way. If you do not know how to swim, you can still float and stretch your body in the water and enjoy its therapeutic benefits. You can also do aerobic exercises while holding onto the edge of the pool.

DOES YOUR LIFESTYLE MAXIMIZE YOUR ENERGY?

The energy that you have depends to a large degree on your diet and lifestyle. Not getting enough rest, too much stress, a poor diet, and no exercise are the major factors that lead to energy loss, weight gain, and poor health. Answer this questionnaire to find out whether your lifestyle is making it difficult for your body to get the energy it needs. Write the answer to each question on a piece of paper, then count how many a's, b's, and c's you have. In the key below you can find out what each letter means and how to improve your lifestyle.

How many times a week do you exercise?

a) Three or more
b) Once or twice
c) Never

Do you smoke cigarettes or any other tobacco products?

a) Rarely
b) Sometimes
c) Often

Do you ever experience a shortness of breath?

a) Only after exercise
b) After any physical exertion
c) Most of the time

How many portions of fruits and vegetables, excluding potatoes, do you eat every day?

a) 5 or more
b) 2 to 4
c) 0 or 1

Are you stressed or anxious or feel that you have lost control of your life?

a) Rarely
b) Sometimes
c) Often

How many alcoholic drinks do you consume on average each day?

a) 0–2
b) 3–5
c) More than 6

How do you feel about your weight?

a) About right
b) Could lose 5 to 10 pounds (2 to 5 kilograms)
c) Could lose more than 10 pounds (5 kilograms)

Do you feel relaxed and unflustered?

a) Most of the time
b) Sometimes or often
c) Rarely

Do you get the sleep that you need?

a) Usually
b) Sometimes or often
c) Rarely

Do you ever feel that you cannot be bothered with or lack the motivation to do something that you have planned to do?

a) Rarely
b) Sometimes
c) Often

Do you lie in bed in the morning because you don't want or don't feel able to get up?

a) Rarely
b) Sometimes
c) Often

How many portions of fried food, candy, cakes, and cookies do you consume on average every day?

a) 0–2
b) 3–5
c) More than 6

Do you need caffeine to get going in the morning?

a) Rarely or sometimes
b) Often
c) Every day

Do you feel that you waste your energy on things of no benefit?

a) Rarely
b) Sometimes
c) Often

How often do you take time off to relax and forget your worries?

a) Twice a week at least
b) Once a week or every two weeks
c) Once a month or less

Mostly a's: You are living a healthy lifestyle and should have no problem in finding the energy that you need to do the things you want to do. Make a note of any questions that you did not score well on and watch out for those problems that are holding you back. Keeping your lifestyle healthy is not always easy, especially in times of trouble, and it is always important to take time off to relax properly. Relaxation techniques can be found in Chapter 5. Making sure that your diet is well balanced and boosting your energy with vitamin-rich fruits and vegetables may also help you to maintain good health.

Mostly b's: Although your lifestyle is relatively healthy, there are still a number of ways that it can be improved. Paying a little more attention to your health will increase the quality of your life, giving you the energy for all the things that you want to do. Making sure that you have a well-balanced and healthful diet is an easy way to enhance your health (see Chapter 4). Cutting down on caffeine can also help you maintain your energy levels.

Mostly c's: You need to pay more attention to your health and lifestyle and make some adjustments if you want to increase your energy levels. Regular vigorous exercise can boost your health substantially (see pages 112–118), and making sure that you get enough sleep to recuperate will help rebalance your system (see pages 54–57). Cutting down on alcohol and smoking may also help, especially in the morning, when energy may be particularly hard to find.

THE GROWTH SPURT

Children have growth spurts, especially around puberty, when the body is preparing for reproduction. Youngsters need more food during this period, particularly boys, whose spurts are greater and come slightly later than those of girls. (To convert centimeters to inches, multiply by 2.54.)

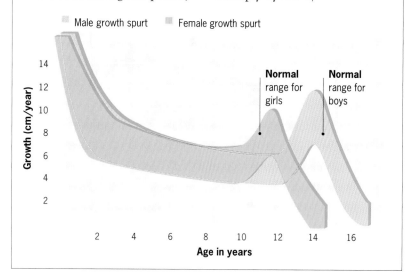

glands, which respond to a number of stimuli. The more important hormones in energy metabolism include thyroxine, insulin, glucagon, and adrenaline.

Thyroxine, produced in the thyroid gland, controls the metabolic rate of energy production. Insulin and glucagon, produced by the pancreas, and adrenaline, produced by the adrenal glands (situated on top of the kidneys), are the two hormones that control the production and use of glucose and glycogen. The latter is synthesized from surplus glucose in the bloodstream and stored in the liver and muscles. When blood-glucose levels need boosting, glycogen is converted back into glucose.

Insulin and glucagon together regulate the amount of glucose in the blood to keep it close to its optimum level. When your blood-glucose level falls, either because more glucose is being used to produce energy or you have not eaten for some time, glucagon stimulates the breakdown of the glycogen reserves within the body into glucose. This breakdown is accelerated when necessary by the action of thyroxine or adrenaline when extra energy is needed.

Insulin has the opposite effect. When your blood-glucose level rises above normal, as it does after eating a meal, insulin stimulates the production of glycogen to mop up the excess, and when your glycogen stores are

THE INFLUENCE OF HORMONES

Hormones are substances that circulate in the bloodstream and act as chemical messengers, carrying signals that control and coordinate the various functions of your body's cells and organs. They are secreted by the

THE ENDOCRINE SYSTEM

The endocrine system is a complex network of hormone-producing glands. The hypothalamus in the brain stimulates the pituitary gland, which in turn regulates most of the other hormones in the body. The pituitary stimulates the adrenals, thyroid, pigment-producing skin cells, and gonads, which control the sex hormones. It also secretes growth hormone, antidiuretic hormone, prolactin, which stimulates the growth and development of the breasts, and oxytocin, which is important during pregnancy.

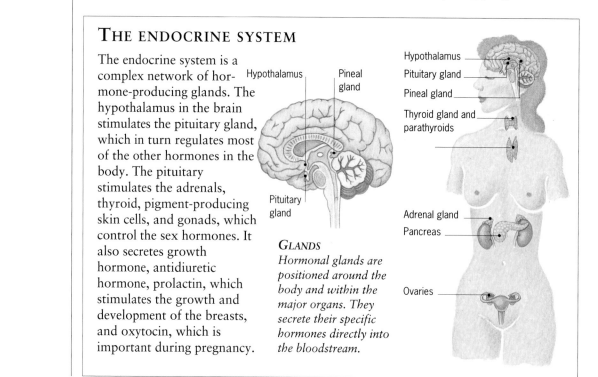

GLANDS
Hormonal glands are positioned around the body and within the major organs. They secrete their specific hormones directly into the bloodstream.

full, it will initiate the conversion of glucose to body fat. It also plays a key role in the production of energy by enabling the transport of glucose into the cells from the bloodstream. Without insulin this process would not be possible.

A temporary low level of blood glucose may occur if you miss a meal. This can make you feel low in energy, irritable, and unable to concentrate, but these symptoms soon disappear when you eat and your blood-glucose level returns to normal.

A serious cause of low blood glucose is the presence of excess insulin in the bloodstream. This can happen to people with insulin-dependent diabetes, a metabolic disorder caused by the failure of the pancreas to produce enough insulin, if they accidentally take too much insulin or fail to eat enough carbohydrates. (Insulin-dependent diabetics routinely inject themselves with insulin, at least once a day, in order to prevent their blood-glucose levels from becoming too high; at the same time they strive to eat enough carbohydrates to prevent glucose levels from becoming too low.) If their glucose levels become dangerously low, this situation can be quickly remedied by taking a sugary food or drink, but if ignored, it can result in unconsciousness.

Hormonal balance plays a major role in vitality. Keeping your body healthy can help you achieve an equilibrium between the chemical hormones being produced by the body and those being used.

Anything, such as exercise, that reduces stress and infection and promotes good sleep will clearly have a beneficial effect on general health and energy levels, especially with increasing age. Both exercise and various forms of relaxation therapy appear to have direct effects on the hormones that influence energy levels.

Researchers at James Cook University in Australia studied the relationship between hormones and mood changes in 11 elite runners and 12 highly trained meditators who were matched for age, sex, and personality. Each performed their specialized activity for 30 minutes, and their hormone changes were then registered over a period of time following the activity. The findings were that both activities stimulated similar hormonal responses, in addition to a general lift in mood. The hormone cortisol, which has been found to be significant in energy

THE HORMONES

The hormones play an important part in the functioning of the human body. If they are out of balance or undergoing a process of change, the body will react differently from the way it is supposed to and will not be able to utilize energy effectively.

LOCATION	HORMONES PRODUCED	EFFECTS
Hypothalamus	Regulating hormones	Regulation of other glands
Pituitary gland	Growth hormone Prolactin	Growth, metabolism Breast development
Brain	Endorphins	Painkilling and relaxation
Pineal gland	Melatonin	Synchronizing of biorhythms
Thyroid glands	Thyroxine	Metabolic rate
Adrenal glands	Adrenaline, noradrenaline Cortisol	Preparation for stress Hormone regulation
Pancreas	Insulin, glucagon	Regulation of blood-sugar level
Ovaries	Estrogen, progesterone	Menstruation, pregnancy, female sexual characteristics
Testes	Testosterone	Male sexual characteristics

function, was higher in most participants at the end of their performance. This suggests that both practices can provide a boost in energy levels, and there is a growing use of meditation, as well as regular exercise, in trying to relieve or eliminate fatigue.

continued on page 28

COSMIC ENERGY FORCES: *The Planets*

The planets have long played a major role in theories of cosmic forces. The Greeks and Romans viewed them as gods and assigned each one a certain power. Mars, for example, was given the role of god of war, and Venus was named the goddess of love. There are nine known planets in our solar system, although some astronomers suspect that there may be more. The planets form the central basis for biodynamic theory, which makes use of their characteristics to understand patterns of nature. The theory is used mostly within an agricultural context.

The Endocrinologist

Specializing in hormone disorders, an endocrinologist can help uncover any hormone or glandular problems that may be affecting your energy levels and preventing you from being active. Endocrinologists can also help with hormone changes.

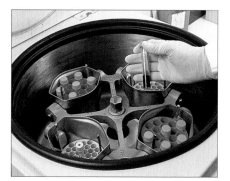

TESTING FOR HORMONE DISORDERS
A number of tests are used to check hormone balance. Some can be performed by an endocrinologist, although others require specialized laboratory analysis.

An endocrinologist investigates problems with the endocrine system—the network of glands involved in the production of hormones and the factors that stimulate them. Because hormones act as chemical messengers, controlling and coordinating virtually every function of the body, any imbalance in this important system can result in a lack of energy, as well as a number of other symptoms of poor health.

Origins

The pituitary gland has been recognized for its importance in brain function since the ancient Greek philosopher Aristotle proposed that a serum was emitted from the gland, influencing body processes. However, endocrinology has only recently become more fully understood. Guesses throughout the 19th century that the source of diabetes lay in the pancreas led to the discovery of glycogen by Claude Bernard in the 1850s, although insulin was not discovered until the 1920s by two Canadian physiologists, Frederick Banting and Charles Best. The first hormone to be isolated was secretin, discovered in 1902 by English physicians William Bayliss and Ernest Starling.

Much of the work done by the American surgeon Harvey Cushing, who greatly advanced neurosurgery in the 1930s, focused on the pituitary gland. He suggested that "the pituitary is the conductor of the endocrine orchestra," paving the way for further hormone research and developments in treatment.

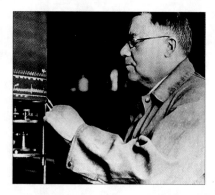

DR. WALTER CANNON
Working as a doctor in the United States in the 1930s, Cannon made great advances in the understanding of hormones and the mental state. His results and conclusions marked a major breakthrough in endocrinology.

What qualifications does an endocrinologist have?
An endocrinologist first trains as a doctor in an accredited medical school and, after serving an internship, does specialized training for another year in endocrinology.

When are patients referred to an endocrinologist?
A primary care physician will refer a patient to an endocrinologist if there is sufficient reason to suspect a problem with the hormone system. Common symptoms that may suggest an endocrine disorder include chronic fatigue, inexplicable weight change, depression, continuous anxiety or mood swings, changes in skin and hair condition, unusual diarrhea or constipation, menstrual disorders, increased urinary output, and swelling of glands, particularly those located in the neck. The doctor will usually eliminate more common or simpler disorders before referring a patient to an endocrinologist.

What will take place during a consultation?
An endocrinologist will order blood and urine tests to examine the levels of different hormones in the system. The results should reveal any discrepancies, which can then be treated. The treatment may be given by the endocrinologist, but sometimes the patient is referred back to his or her own doctor with the test results for further care. Other symptoms and your health history,

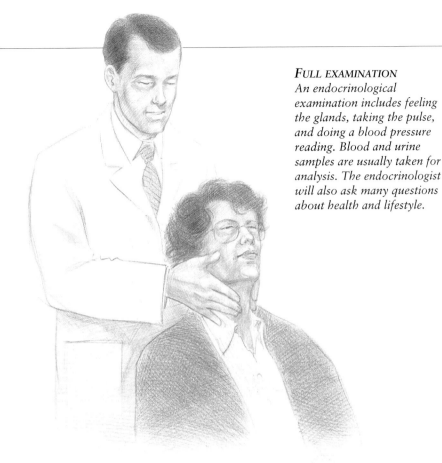

FULL EXAMINATION
An endocrinological examination includes feeling the glands, taking the pulse, and doing a blood pressure reading. Blood and urine samples are usually taken for analysis. The endocrinologist will also ask many questions about health and lifestyle.

lead to a drain on energy levels and an inability to live a normal life. The efficient working of the thyroid gland is essential for retaining healthy metabolic function, and an endocrinologist can effectively diagnose and treat imbalances and restore health and vitality. Insulin disorders causing diabetes mellitus prevent glucose from being converted into energy, and insulin injections or dietary measures can help normalize the energy balance. Hormones affecting the brain can also be rebalanced, including those that cause depression, anxiety, and other debilitating psychological conditions that can sap a person's vitality and motivation.

Where does an endocrinologist practice?

Most are associated with endo-crinology departments in larger hospitals, although smaller hospitals that specialize in reproductive, digestive, or psychological disorders also have endocrinology units to help with hormonal disorders.

including emotional health, will be taken into consideration when deciding on the treatment, which may involve hormone replacement drugs, lifestyle changes, dietary measures, and other treatments.

What are the most common conditions an endocrinologist treats?

Thyroid disorders and diabetes are common problems that need to be treated by an endocrinologist. An analysis of the hypothalamus-pituitary system is also carried out on anyone who has depressed energy levels. The hypothalamus and the pituitary gland, located at the base of the brain, play major roles in all hormone production.

Some endocrinologists specialize in locating hormonal problems that involve low energy and related disorders, such as chronic fatigue syndrome, or myalgic encephalo-myelitis (see pages 150–153).

Many other common hormonal problems, such as menstrual disorders, imbalances caused by menopause, and prostate problems, are usually treated by a specialist in the reproductive organs.

How can an endocrinologist help to boost energy levels?

Hormonal complications come in a variety of forms, almost all of which

WHAT YOU CAN DO AT HOME

Some hormone problems can be countered at home by through dietary measures. Several minerals and vitamins can play key roles in keeping you feeling normal through difficult hormonal changes.

For example, many people have a problem maintaining their sex drive after the hormonal changes that occur in middle age, and this affects their sense of well-being and their energy levels. This can be countered to some extent with a healthful and balanced diet that provides all the necessary nutrients. Zinc levels are considered particularly important in sexual activity; when zinc levels are low, blood histamine levels are also low, which may make it more difficult to reach orgasm. Because refining processes remove 80 percent of the zinc content from cereals and grains, it is important to choose

whole-grain or fortified cereals and other foods that keep zinc intake high. Good sources include oysters, clams, sardines, and other seafood, seeds, nuts, and red meat.

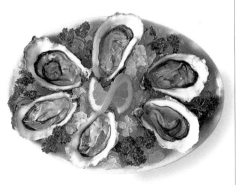

THE ULTIMATE APHRODISIAC
The ancient Greeks celebrated oysters for their aphrodisiac qualities, and the bivalve's reputation remains to this day. Oysters contain high levels of important nutrients that support a good sex life.

EFFECTS OF LOW ENERGY

Low energy can produce the following effects:

► *Inactivity*
► *Intolerance to cold*
► *Irritability*
► *Depression or anxiety*
► *Poor skin and hair condition*
► *Tendency to illness*

CULTURAL FACTORS
Living conditions and lifestyles in different cultures produce different energy demands. This woman, carrying her baby as she works, is also responsible for breast-feeding the infant and so will need a greater number of calories in her diet than a woman of similar age in a leisured society.

HORMONAL CHANGES

Hormonal changes, which affect everyone throughout life, sometimes have serious effects on metabolism and energy levels. Most changes occur as the body alters with age, such as at menopause. However, many changes cannot be explained and may result from illness or stress or occur for no apparent reason at all. The endocrine system—the network of glands that releases hormones into the bloodstream—may be affected by a number of factors, including emotional and mental processes.

The hormone condition most often linked with fatigue is thyroid disease, or a change in production of the hormone thyroxine, which is needed to stimulate metabolism. Insufficient thyroxine, which causes hypothyroidism or myxedema, can lead to lethargy, weight gain, and muscular problems and can also slow thinking and mental development in children. It can be treated easily with thyroid hormone replacement.

The adrenal glands are responsible for the production of adrenaline, the hormone that causes blood to flow faster and the body to respond quickly to challenging situations. An excess of adrenaline and its related hormone, noradrenaline, results in high blood pressure, increased activity, anxiety, and in the long run, fatigue.

Another important hormone that influences energy levels is cortisol. This is released by the adrenal cortex and regulated by a complicated feedback mechanism involving both the hypothalamus and the pituitary gland. Low levels of cortisol can result in

profound lethargy, which is reversible only with hormone replacement treatment.

Hormones concerned with reproduction can also cause energy imbalances. Changes in hormone levels during the menstrual cycle and also during menopause can greatly affect energy levels. Pregnancy brings about probably the greatest changes in hormones experienced in a woman's life. Male hormones, especially testosterone, can play a major role in a man's energy levels.

GENETIC FACTORS

Genetics may be a factor in how much energy some people have. Abnormalities that can influence a person's energy may be present at birth but not become apparent until middle or old age. Common disorders that have a pronounced effect on metabolism and thus energy expenditure, and in which there is probably some genetic predisposition, include diabetes mellitus and thyroid disease. The Pima Indians of North America, who are predisposed to develop diabetes, are an example of this genetic factor.

CULTURAL FACTORS

Unused food energy is usually stored as fat, and the fat stores in people differ widely throughout the world, depending on food supply and climate. In modern societies, particularly those in highly developed countries that have abundant food and labor-saving devices, there is a tendency toward being overweight. Energy levels are greatly affected by fat levels because being overweight lowers mobility and greatly increases the likelihood of energy-draining conditions such as diabetes, hypertension, heart disease, arthritis, and other illnesses.

Energy expenditure is also modified by social customs and by how an individual is brought up. Psychological, social, and cultural factors, including race and religion, influence diet and hence individual energy expenditure. Different cultures have traditional ways of preparing and eating food that can make a great impact on energy and health. The typical diet in North America is dominated by fried foods, although more healthful cooking approaches are taking hold. It is estimated that 13 percent of men and 16 percent of women are obese, and a huge number—43 percent of men and some 24 percent of women—are overweight, which causes many energy and health problems.

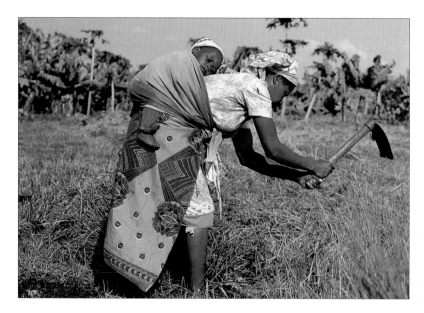

WOMEN AND ENERGY

Throughout life women tend to experience more ups and downs in their energy levels than men, mainly because of the hormonal changes associated with menstruation and pregnancy.

Undergoing complicated hormonal changes every month with menstruation, women often find themselves feeling out of sorts and fatigued for no apparent reason. Realizing and understanding the difficulties can allow you to boost your energy by maintaining a balanced diet, exercising properly, and taking precautions to prevent draining your energy during the times when you need it most.

PREMENSTRUAL SYNDROME

The hormonal changes associated with the menstrual cycle can cause a range of symptoms, including food cravings, behavioral and mood changes, irritability, tenderness of the breasts, swelling of the legs and abdomen, weight gain (from water retention), skin outbreaks, headaches, and lack of energy.

The symptoms occur between eight and two days before menstruation begins and are known collectively as premenstrual syndrome

(PMS). Women vary considerably in the number and severity of their PMS symptoms; lack of energy seems to be common.

One of the first descriptions of PMS was put forth in 1937 by three doctors in London who reported on physical and emotional responses to menstruation in the *Journal of Hygiene*. In their detailed study of 167 women, they found that fatigue and lack of energy were the most frequently reported symptoms. Why women should lack energy at this time is still unknown, but it is likely

DID YOU KNOW?

There have been several court cases that have cited PMS as the cause for a defendant's behavior. These claims have had varying degrees of success in helping defendants' cases, but no one has yet been acquitted on the grounds of PMS.

ENERGY BOOST

Invite a friend for dinner and prepare one of your favorite dishes. Having a good chat over a meal is an excellent way to relieve pressure and boost good feelings.

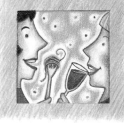

FEMALE REPRODUCTIVE SYSTEM

The main function of the female reproductive system is to provide ova and a safe, comfortable, and healthy environment for their growth and development. The human female is fertile all year round, releasing an ovum on average every 28 days. To regulate this complex system, several hormones are produced at different times throughout the menstrual cycle, and they affect physical and emotional balance.

FEMALE HORMONES
Estrogen and progesterone, which prepare the body for pregnancy, peak around the time of ovulation. They are the most important female hormones.

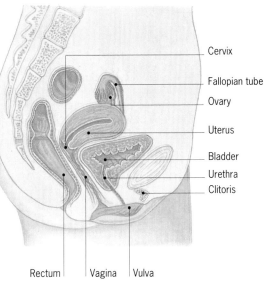

Cervix
Fallopian tube
Ovary
Uterus
Bladder
Urethra
Clitoris

Rectum | Vagina | Vulva

COSMIC ENERGY FORCES: *The Stars*

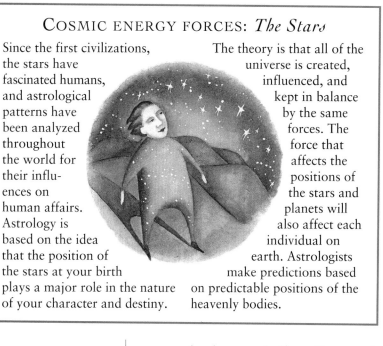

Since the first civilizations, the stars have fascinated humans, and astrological patterns have been analyzed throughout the world for their influences on human affairs. Astrology is based on the idea that the position of the stars at your birth plays a major role in the nature of your character and destiny.

The theory is that all of the universe is created, influenced, and kept in balance by the same forces. The force that affects the positions of the stars and planets will also affect each individual on earth. Astrologers make predictions based on predictable positions of the heavenly bodies.

primrose, flaxseeds, and black currant seeds, may also help, although tests have been inconclusive. Soy products such as tofu are definitely beneficial because they help to balance estrogen in the system.

In general, it is better to avoid foods and beverages that contain caffeine or refined sugar and also highly salted foods, which increase water retention. Regular exercise is very helpful in reducing symptoms of PMS. Aerobic exercise, in particular, increases the brain's production of endorphins, substances that lift mood.

Although hormone treatment, usually with progesterone, has been used to restore hormonal balance and reduce the effects of PMS, studies on its effectiveness have been inconsistent. Diet and lifestyle changes seem to be more effective. Keep in mind that the fatigue associated with PMS can be aggravated by stress and concerns about being unable to do as much as usual. Remind yourself to avoid demanding situations in the week before your period.

PREGNANCY

The female body undergoes enormous changes during pregnancy. As the fetus grows, conspicuous changes take place in virtually every system of the mother. The uterine enlarges, changing both its shape and function; the breasts become larger; blood volume increases by 30 percent; and body weight and respiratory activity also

connected to hormonal effects. Recent evidence suggests that a principal cause of premenstrual fatigue is related to a lowering of progesterone levels and an increase in estrogen in combination with other factors.

A number of nutritional imbalances may also occur, including disturbances of iron metabolism and changes in vitamin levels in the body. Supplements of vitamin B_6 and magnesium have been found very helpful in some cases of PMS, as have supplements of vitamin E. Taking gamma linolenic acid (GLA), a constituent of the oils of evening

PMS AND MOOD SWINGS

The physical changes involved in the menstrual cycle are well documented, but the emotional impact of all the hormonal changes has been more difficult to gauge. Some of the findings suggested by research are shown below.

■ Sexual interest　■ Energy　Happiness

■ Irritability　Physical complaints　■ Unhappiness

Ovulation

Ovulation

| 1 | 7 | 14 | 21 | 28 |

28-day cycle

| 1 | 7 | 14 | 21 | 28 |

28-day cycle

POSITIVE MOODS
The more positive mood swings occur close to the time of ovulation, when estrogen and progesterone levels are at their highest.

NEGATIVE MOODS
Negative mood swings come to the forefront before, during, and immediately after menstruation, possibly contributing to PMS.

VITAMINS AND MINERALS FOR PREGNANCY

Obtaining sufficient vitamins and minerals is vital to the healthy development of a fetus, but the ones below are especially important. Doctors also advise taking folic acid supplements prior to pregnancy and during the first 12 weeks.

NUTRIENT	USES	SOURCES
Protein	Provides the building blocks of all body tissue.	Meat, fish, dairy products, beans, soy products
Calcium	Builds strong bones and teeth.	Dairy products, sardines with bones, dark greens
Vitamin C	Promotes iron absorption; strengthens blood cells.	Citrus fruits, berries, peppers, broccoli
Iron	Transfers and transports oxygen.	Red meat, fish, beans, dark leafy greens, beans
Vitamin A	Promotes cell growth and development.	Dairy products, eggs, fish, fruit, vegetables
Vitamins B_1, B_2, B_3, and B_6	Metabolize carbohydrates.	Whole grains, lean meats, poultry, beans
Folic acid	Builds DNA, RNA, and central nervous system.	Fortified cereals, liver, spinach, broccoli, beans
Vitamin D	Promotes absorption of calcium and phosphorus.	Oily fish, eggs, dairy products
Vitamin E	Maintains red blood cells; deficiency can lead to miscarriage.	Wheat germ, eggs, dark leafy greens, nuts, seeds, vegetable oils
Phosphorus	Promotes calcium absorption and metabolism.	Meat, fish, egg yolks, dairy products, beans

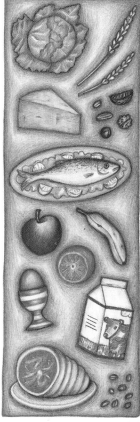

increase. Because of these physical changes, the mother could find herself lacking in energy if she doesn't pay close attention to her diet and get sufficient rest. Most women need to add about 300 calories and 10 grams of protein a day to their diet to support normal fetal growth, especially during the last two trimesters. (Doubling food intake is not recommended, as this can lead to excessive weight gain and accompanying problems.) Increasing calcium intake is also important. If the mother does not take in sufficient calcium, it will be gathered from her bones to make sure that calcification of the fetal bones occurs correctly.

The fetus can be adversely affected by alcohol and nicotine, and these should be avoided. Studies show that women who have even one or two drinks a day tend to have undersized babies. Smoking increases the risk of miscarriage and low birth weight. Many medicines, both over-the-counter and prescription, can have a harmful effect; none should be taken without a doctor's prescription or advice. Also, hot baths and saunas may reduce a mother's energy levels.

Keeping fit during pregnancy is of great importance, and although excessive energy expenditure and stress on the joints should be avoided, moderate exercise throughout pregnancy will be beneficial. Improved energy metabolism and aerobic and muscular fitness from regular exercise should lead to easier labor and quicker postnatal recovery.

continued on page 34

NATURAL CHILDBIRTH

In the mid-20th century, most women in North America had their babies in hospitals, lying flat on their backs (the most difficult position for pushing the baby), usually with full technological intervention, which might include drugs to induce strong uterine contractions, anesthesia, and the use of forceps. In the 1960s a trend to return to natural childbirth emerged. This approach has the woman sitting, rather than lying down, and using special breathing techniques instead of anesthesia to control pain. There has also been a growing movement toward the use of midwives.

FOODS TO AVOID DURING PREGNANCY

Food poisoning from toxoplasmosis or listeriosis can lead to miscarriage or impaired development of the fetus. Foods to avoid include:

► *Raw or incompletely cooked meat, particularly hamburger and poultry*

► *Soft cheeses*

► *Raw eggs*

► *Raw fish*

Pregnancy

The nine months of pregnancy take a woman through a variety of physical and emotional phases. Energy levels rise and fall with the demands of fetal growth and changes in the woman's hormones. A healthy diet, rest, and exercise are essential.

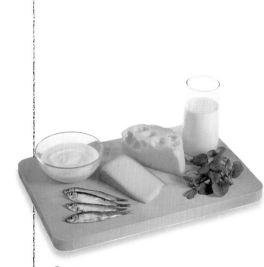

CALCIUM IN THE DIET
A pregnant woman needs 1,200 milligrams of calcium a day, which is about 50 percent more than normal. The foods richest in calcium are dairy products like milk, yogurt, and cheese. Other good sources include canned sardines with bones, watercress and other dark green vegetables, and tofu.

Understanding and adapting to the changes your body is going through is one of the keys to keeping up your energy during pregnancy. You will have to make a few adjustments in your diet, exercise, and rest routines.

Supplements of iron and folate are recommended for pregnant women. Discuss with your doctor the amounts that would be appropriate and the possible need for other supplements as well. Extra vitamin A should be avoided because in high doses it can cause birth defects. However, its precursor, beta carotene, is plentiful in fruits and vegetables, especially yellow and orange varieties.

Rest plays an important part in giving your body the energy it needs to help the baby develop normally. Biologically, the demands of your baby will be met at your expense, so if you feel tired, it may be that your resources have been drained and your body is simply telling you to rest. Making time to take it easy and avoiding stressful situations as much as possible can help you retain high energy levels, while encouraging the healthy growth of your baby.

Exercise also plays a role in good health care during pregnancy; maintaining a balance of rest and exercise is the best strategy.

TRIMESTER 1: 0–12 WEEKS

During the first trimester the body is adjusting to its new condition and major hormonal upheavals. The metabolic rate rises between 10 and 25 percent because of the energy needed for the baby's growth and for the changes in your own body. You probably will not gain weight during this period and may even lose a little. It is common to become tired easily, because much of your energy is focused on the growing fetus.

Morning sickness—nausea and vomiting that may actually occur any time during the day—is a problem for many women during the first trimester. Some measures that can help relieve it include eating smaller and more frequent meals, sipping ginger ale or ginger tea, avoiding spicy and fried foods, and eating crackers or dry toast before getting out of bed in

the morning. In clinical studies, many women have obtained relief with supplements of vitamin B$_6$ or a combined supplement of vitamins C and K. Consult with your doctor about the most effective dosage.

▶ *Increase your intake of protein- and calcium-rich foods.*

▶ *Drink more fluids.*

▶ *Eliminate alcohol and nicotine and reduce consumpton of caffeine.*

▶ *Eat smaller, more frequent meals, particularly if you suffer morning sickness.*

▶ *Wear a good supportive bra to ease tenderness in the breasts.*

DRINKING MORE FLUIDS
Keep up your fluid intake by keeping a bottle of mineral water or fruit juice handy so that you can take a sip whenever you need it.

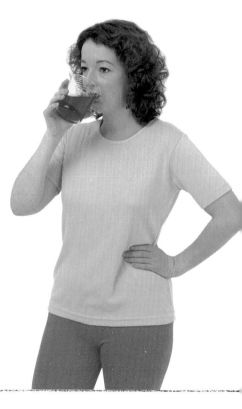

TRIMESTER 2: 13–28 WEEKS

This is the period when you start to feel more comfortable with being pregnant. The major hormonal changes will have taken place, but the metabolic rate will remain high, and it is essential that you eat well. A woman who was an ideal weight before conceiving should gain an average of one pound a week during this and the last trimester; underweight women should gain slightly more, overweight women a little less. You may experience constipation and other digestive complaints.

▶ *Lessen backache by maintaining good posture.*

▶ *Consume lots of fluids and fiber to prevent constipation, hemorrhoids, and diarrhea.*

▶ *Keep meals small to deal with heartburn and crowding of the stomach and intestines.*

▶ *Take time to relax.*

Shoulders should be held square.

LIFTING POSTURE
When lifting, bend your knees and use your legs—not your back and shoulders—to lift the object.

Buttocks should be tucked in.

Use both hands to lift heavy objects.

STANDING POSTURE
It is easy to slip into a poor posture when you are pregnant to compensate for the extra weight in front. Bad posture can lead to backache and prevent ease of movement.

Knees should be slightly bent

Feet should be shoulder width apart.

TRIMESTER 3: 29 WEEKS–DELIVERY

During the third trimester you may find it difficult to get a good night's sleep because of the baby's movements, your own general discomfort, and the need to urinate frequently. Your breathing may become shallower because of restricted movement of the diaphragm, leaving you feeling breathless and low in energy. You may also experience leg cramps and increased fluid retention; these are common, brought on by changes in the body's electrolyte balance.

▶ *It may be difficult to sleep for long periods, so take naps during the day.*

▶ *Try to resist urges to do excessive cleaning and decorating; you will need your energy for childbirth.*

▶ *Relieve water retention problems by sitting down regularly and putting your feet up to increase circulation.*

▶ *Relieve discomfort in your chest by propping yourself up with cushions.*

▶ *Increase intake of fluids and fruits and vegetables.*

RESTING POSITIONS
The best positions when lying down are on the side and the back. Do not lie flat on your back, however, as this may lead to blood flow problems around your pelvis and abdomen (see below). Keep extra cushions and pillows at hand for creating more comfort.

Raise your top knee with a cushion or pillow.

FOOD CRAVINGS

Pregnant women often crave particular foods, some of which they would not normally favor. Bananas, pickles, and ice cream are common examples. The phenomenon is believed to be the result of hormonal changes, which unbalance the system, although it may sometimes be due to the body demanding certain nutrients. It is mostly harmless to give in to cravings, especially if the foods are nutritionally wholesome, although you should not eat too many fatty foods. A very rare condition known as pica occurs when pregnant women have a peculiar desire for nonfood substances, such as coal, plaster, or clay. This is a more serious problem, and you should see a doctor if you find yourself wanting nonfoods.

ENDOMETRIOSIS

Endometriosis occurs when pieces of the endometrium, which lines the uterus, attach to other pelvic structures, such as the ovaries and fallopian tubes. The renegade tissue bleeds just like the uterus during menstruation, and with no place for the blood to go, the tissue becomes swollen and inflamed.

Pain in the pelvic area, especially around the time of menstruation, and unexplained fatigue are the most frequent symptoms. Experiencing pain during intercourse and bowel movements is also common. In many cases, however, the condition is symptomless, and as yet no causes for it are known.

Endometriosis occurs usually between the ages of 25 and 40 and is relatively common. Severe endometriosis can interfere with fertility and cause ovarian dysfunction; it is estimated that between 30 and 40 percent of cases result in some degree of infertility.

MENOPAUSE

Menopause, the cessation of menstruation, occurs around age 50, although it can happen anytime between 40 and 60 and occasionally as early as 28. There is usually a period of about two years from the time of the first symptoms until menstruation finally ends. A variety of symptoms characterizes menopause, including mood swings, hot flashes, insomnia, vaginal dryness, and memory problems. In addition, the risk of osteoporosis and heart disease greatly increase at this time. Since women in the Western world now live well past 50, it is important that energy disturbances and other problems of menopause be rectified.

One approach is hormonal replacement therapy (HRT)—low doses of estrogen and progesterone—to protect against osteoporosis and heart disease. Natural ways of dealing with menopause include eating tofu and other soy products for their phytoestrogens and taking additional calcium and doing weight-bearing exercises to maintain bone mass.

CAUSES OF CANDIDIASIS

Candidiasis, or vaginal thrush, is a fungal infection that can invade the vaginal area when the body's defenses are lowered. Its causes include:

► *A course of antibiotics, which kills the body's natural protective bacteria*

► *Hormonal changes due to pregnancy or taking the contraceptive pill or steroids, for example*

► *Restricted air circulation from tight or synthetic clothing*

► *Conditions that encourage fungal growth, such as hot, damp weather*

COMMON CAUSES OF FATIGUE

Candidiasis, a fungal infection of the vaginal area, can have a detrimental effect on energy. Cystitis, an inflammation of the bladder, is another energy drainer. It may be caused by bacteria that live in the intestines or by chlamydia, a sexually transmitted organism that invades the bladder through the urethra.

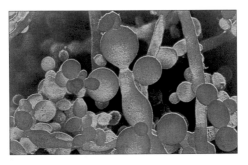

CANDIDA
The electromicrograph shown here depicts the tiny growth of cells that cause the irritation and discomfort of candidiasis.

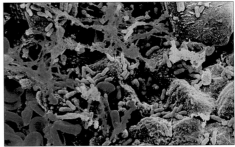

CYSTITIS
This electromicrograph shows the bladder lining ruptured by bacteria (green), causing red blood cells to escape into the urine.

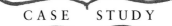
A Fatigued Lawyer

Unexplained pelvic pain and loss of energy, especially before and after menstruation, may be signs of endometriosis. With this condition, pieces of the endometrium (uterus lining) migrate to other parts of the pelvis and bleed during menstruation just as the uterus does. A few treatments for it are available. The problem often disappears with pregnancy.

Esther is 32 years old and makes a good, though stressful, living as a lawyer. She was looking forward to becoming pregnant when she developed pain in her lower abdomen about six months ago. It has gradually become a dragging, incapacitating pain that usually begins four days before her menstrual period and lasts until three days after it ends. Sex with her husband, Mark, has also became painful, and the condition has begun to interfere with her work, affecting her concentration and energy levels. Esther has not been able to become pregnant, and this is causing her further anxiety. Fearing a serious problem with her reproductive system, she makes an appointment with her gynecologist.

WHAT SHOULD ESTHER DO?

The problem must be investigated thoroughly, and Esther's physician may have to do several tests in addition to a full pelvic examination. If the doctor suspects endometriosis and has excluded other possible causes, she may do a laparoscopic procedure—insertion of a viewing instrument into the abdominal cavity through a small incision near the navel—to confirm the diagnosis. To remedy the condition, Esther may be prescribed an oral contraceptive for a few months, which will reduce the flow of her periods and allow her body to destroy the abnormal tissue. If adhesions have occurred in any of her abdominal organs, she may need surgery to remove the adhesions.

Action Plan

HEALTH
Seek the cause of chronic pain. Ignoring a problem can allow it become worse and perhaps lead to more serious consequences.

LIFESTYLE
Prioritize time and focus on what is really important. Do not try to do too much at once.

SELF-HELP
Try a hot bath or heating pad to relieve abdominal pain. Massaging the area may also help. Take valerian extract or capsules to relieve cramps. Eat soy and other beans for their plant estrogens.

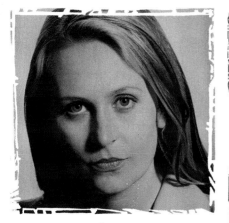

LIFESTYLE
Trying to fit too much into your life can increase stress and cause health problems.

STRESS
Chronic stress can exacerbate pain and contribute to fatigue.

HEALTH
Ignoring physical or emotional problems can take its toll on energy and allow the problems to worsen.

HOW THINGS TURNED OUT FOR ESTHER

Esther was diagnosed with endometriosis and was put on a high-estrogen oral contraceptive for a few months to mimic the hormone levels of pregnancy (endometriosis disappears when a woman is not ovulating). Within six months of completing treatment, she became pregnant. Although stress was not the cause of Esther's problem, she and Mark have decided to change their lifestyle so that she can stay home for a few years after the baby arrives.

MEN AND ENERGY

Although men do not undergo the complex hormonal fluctuations that women do, their energy levels are known to vacillate with changes in testosterone production and age.

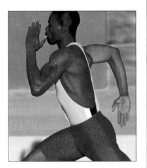

TESTOSTERONE
The hormone that motivates action, drive, and athletic performance, testosterone can also contribute to aggression.

In general, men have a higher metabolic rate than women do and higher energy levels, although they usually have less energy reserved as fat. This is because men have greater amounts of striated muscle and less layered fat on their bodies. Major fluctuations in male energy levels occur during puberty, when the testes begin to produce the hormone testosterone; as men age and testosterone levels decrease; and as a result of using alcohol and drugs.

TESTOSTERONE

Testosterone, the hormone that stimulates the development of the male primary sexual characteristics, is responsible for the big spurt in growth that accompanies puberty. During this period the dietary needs of a boy rise as he gains height and weight and his sexual organs mature. The energy value of food becomes increasingly important. Teenage boys commonly suffer from fatigue due to poor nutrition, and making sure that their diet is high in protein, carbohydrates, and essential nutrients is crucial.

Testosterone has long been considered the energy hormone for its role in encouraging activity, drive, and aggression in men. This hormone has an anabolic, or restorative, effect on body tissues, especially bone marrow and skeletal muscles. This means that if testosterone levels alter, a man may suffer from loss of energy, fatigue, and impotence.

Testosterone levels begin to decline after men reach the age of 50, while estrogen has a tendency to increase. This process often leads to a general loss of energy and a decline in activity.

Testosterone and illness

Testosterone levels are known to drop during a variety of illnesses, including kidney disease and liver cirrhosis, and also as a result of stress, surgery, infection, or a head injury. Low testosterone levels may also be found in patients who have nonspecific illness and low energy, although the reasons are poorly understood and the condition is almost certainly a secondary phenomenon. Low testosterone production may be caused by a high intake of alcohol or certain drugs, leading to testicular atrophy or to other hormonal changes. There are possible benefits of testosterone replacement, although treatments have not been formalized and, to some extent, remain controversial.

PROSTATE PROBLEMS

The prostate is a small, chestnut-sized gland responsible for the production of the seminal fluids that increase the motility of sperm during ejaculation and the secretions that keep the urethra moist and prevent infec-

---

MALE REPRODUCTIVE SYSTEM

The male reproductive system centers on the testicles and penis. The former produce the male gamete (sperm) and the hormone testosterone, responsible for the male characteristics. The penis is used to place the sperm within the reproductive tract of the female for fertilization of her ovum.

PROSTATE GLAND
The prostate gland is responsible for releasing lubricating fluids into the urethra. It grows larger as a result of the hormonal changes associated with aging.

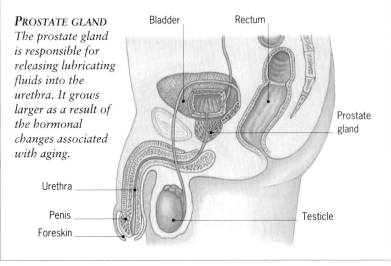

Bladder

Rectum

Prostate gland

Urethra

Penis

Foreskin

Testicle

Impotence

About 10 percent of all men suffer from impotence, most cases arising after the age of 40, when the body slows down with age. Keeping the body fit and healthy is the best measure to counter impotence and enjoy a normal sex life.

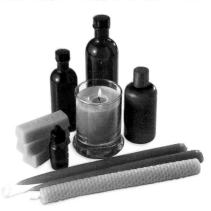

APHRODISIAC MASSAGE OILS
Certain aromatherapy oils have been found to raise libido and levels of sexual stimulation; they include patchouli, rose, jasmine, sandalwood, and ylang-ylang. Mix 5 drops of one of these essential oils with 25 milliliters of massage oil to make enough for a full-body massage.

Impotence is defined as the inability to get or sustain an erection sufficient for sexual intercourse 75 percent of the time. Most men experience a weakening of their erection as they grow older, and they become progressively less able to perform sex as often as they used to. Psychological stresses like anxiety or depression may contribute to impotence, but studies have shown that most cases are due to an underlying disease or the medications used to treat it, as well as lifestyle factors. Damage to the penis can also cause impotence but is less common. One good way to deal with impotence is with relaxation methods (see below).

THE BENEFITS OF RELAXATION

Relaxation is known to play an important role in learning to live with impotence. Taking the pressure off your own performance and concentrating on pleasing your partner can be a successful method for relaxing yourself and allowing your body to react naturally.

▶ *Talking over the issue with your partner so that she can understand your problems can help her to help you.*

▶ *Relaxing and taking the time to address the problem and work with it is a crucial element.*

▶ *Aromatherapy massage oils may aid in achieving relaxation; mood music may also be helpful.*

LIFESTYLE TIPS

A healthy lifestyle can improve your sex life. Researchers have found the following links:

▶*Limit alcohol intake. Alcohol is a depressant that slows down the body's responses to stimulants, limiting a man's ability to get and sustain an erection. It also decreases testosterone production, which is linked to lowered libido.*

▶ *Eat foods rich in zinc—yogurt, shellfish, poultry, whole-grain and fortified cereals, wheat germ, and vegetables. Zinc is essential to good reproductive health.*

▶ *Eat less saturated fat and maintain a normal weight. Fat slows blood circulation and contributes to blockages in the arteries; it also predisposes a person to diabetes, a leading cause of impotence.*

▶ *Give up smoking. It is a major factor in impotence, causing blockages in the arteries that prevent blood from entering the penis.*

▶ *Exercise regularly. According to research, a fitter lifestyle makes you better able to enjoy sex,*

"Aphrodisiacs," such as oysters and other shellfish, provide important minerals.

Relaxation is one key to tackling impotence problems.

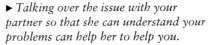

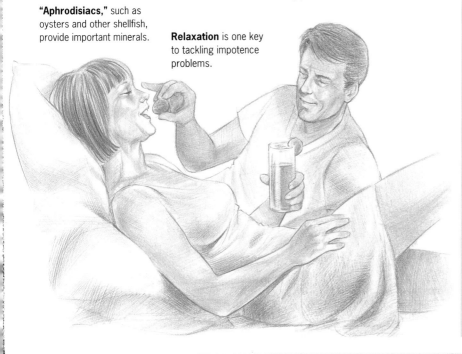

ENERGY BOOST

Bringing a piece of nature inside can add natural energy to a room and in turn boost mental energy. If it is winter, a few twigs and branches, perhaps with pine or fir cones, can enliven the atmosphere. According to Norse and Saxon mythology, the logs and branches brought in at Christmas come from the idea of the Tree of Life, which is said to support the earth, heaven, and hell. You can combine them in a display with evergreen sprigs, such as holly, a fertility and life-bringing tradition from ancient Mesopotamia.

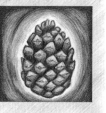

FOODS FOR PROSTATE PROBLEMS
Many men find relief from prostate trouble by eating foods rich in zinc, vitamin E, and vitamin B$_6$. All three are found in nuts and seeds. Zinc can also be found in shellfish, red meat, and whole grains. Vitamin E is plentiful in wheat germ and vegetable oils. Vitamin B$_6$ is available from bananas, vegetables, whole grains, and liver.

tion. It is located at the base of the bladder and surrounds the top part of the urethra. The position of the prostate means that any problems it incurs can cause discomfort in the urinary system.

By far the most common problem is an enlarged prostate, which occurs in most men over the age of 45. The enlargement may or may not cause symptoms. Other, less common conditions include cancer of the prostate and prostatitis—a bacterial infection. All of these conditions can be diagnosed and treated only by a doctor.

Enlarged prostate

Enlargement of the prostate, also known as benign prostatic hypertrophy (BPH), occurs as the body ages. It is not known exactly what causes the problem, but it may be linked to the depletion of testosterone and an increase in other hormones, such as estrogen, which can occur any time after age 40.

As the prostate grows, it puts pressure on the bladder and obstructs the passage of urine, often causing a need to urinate more frequently, especially during the night. This can severely disrupt sleep patterns and lead to fatigue during the day. The condition can eventually cause chronic outflow obstruction, leading to a deterioration of kidney function and an increase of urea in the bloodstream, both of which are potentially serious problems.

The hormone prolactin is believed to antagonize the situation further by encouraging more testosterone to be taken up by the prostate and increasing the synthesis of dihydrotestosterone. Since prolactin levels are increased by alcohol and stress, cutting down on alcohol and taking measures to reduce stress can be beneficial. There are drugs that reduce prolactin levels, but many of them are known to have side effects.

Some doctors and alternative practitioners recommend a diet high in zinc and vitamin B$_6$ to reduce prolactin levels in a more natural way. Other dietary measures recommended for an enlarged prostate include eating more soy products, such as tofu; increasing intake of essential fatty acids and vitamin E, found in flaxseeds, nuts, seeds, and such vegetable oils as canola and corn; and reducing foods that are high in saturated fats and cholesterol.

Saw palmetto extract has also been used to relieve symptoms of an enlarged prostate, but it should be taken only under the supervision of a doctor, as it may interfere with other drugs used to treat BPH. (Health Canada permits the sale of saw palmetto only as a diuretic, not for treating BPH.)

DID YOU KNOW?

Tomatoes (also red grapefruit, watermelon, and berries) contain a pigment called lycopene, which may help prevent prostate cancer. Cooking releases more of the lycopene in tomatoes, so tomato sauces and soups may be especially beneficial.

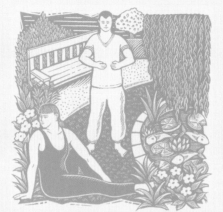

CHAPTER 2

THE ENERGY ALL AROUND US

We are constantly being bombarded by energy—from sunlight and color to sound and electromagnetism. These forces can have both positive and negative effects on us, and many have been harnessed by both orthodox and alternative medicine to improve our energy levels and all-round health.

LIGHT AND COLOR

Light and the associated forces of color and heat are powerful forms of energy that affect our lives in many ways. They have many uses in both conventional and alternative health care.

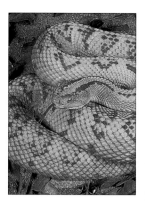

ANIMAL INSIGHT
Many creatures are aware of energy wavelengths other than those that humans can sense. Bees and butterflies, for instance, see UV light, while rattlesnakes detect specific infrared waves through their skin.

Light, color, and heat energy are forms of electromagnetic radiation. They are utilized in conventional medicine, for example, in the form of X-rays and radiotherapy, and in complementary approaches, such as light therapy.

LIGHT AND COLOR

We are consciously aware of only a narrow band of wavelengths in the middle of the electromagnetic spectrum. We see light (the visible spectrum) and we feel heat (infrared waves), and we observe that our skins are tanned by ultraviolet light. Although we cannot directly sense wavelengths above and below this spectrum, they can be detected by instruments, and they often affect our bodies and health in subtle ways.

Different wavelengths of visible light are seen as different colors—violet, blue, green, yellow, orange, and red. These are the rainbow colors that make up the visible spectrum. When white light falls on an object, some wavelengths are absorbed, while others are reflected. If, for instance, only the wavelength that makes blue light is reflected off an object, we see it as blue. If all the wavelengths of light are reflected, we see the object as white. If all the wavelengths are absorbed, however, we see it as black.

LIGHT IN MEDICINE

Various wavelengths of light are employed in conventional medicine. Treatment with light is called phototherapy and includes the use of visible light, ultraviolet (UV) light, and concentrated light beams known as lasers.

Special fluorescent lights are used to treat a form of winter depression called seasonal affective disorder (SAD). This condition mainly affects people who live in northerly latitudes during the winter, when daylight is limited. Sunlight and UV light, often in combination with drugs, are used to treat

THE ELECTROMAGNETIC SPECTRUM

All objects emit heat radiation, which consists of electromagnetic waves. These waves, collectively known as the electromagnetic spectrum, radiate at different wavelengths, some narrow and concentrated, such as X-rays and gamma rays, and others wide and less powerful, such as radio waves. The sun is the most powerful source of electromagnetic radiation. It sends out all forms of radiant energy—not just light and heat. All electromagnetic radiation travels at the speed of light and passes easily through space.

ELECTROMAGNETIC WAVELENGTH
Each group of waves has a different wavelength and carries a different amount of energy. For example, radio waves have a longer wavelength and less energy than shortwave X-rays.

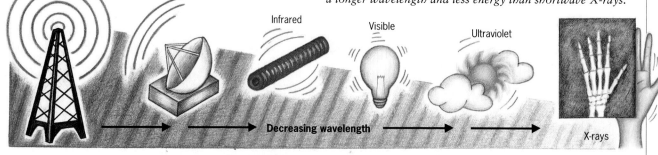

Radio · Microwaves · Infrared · Visible · Ultraviolet

Decreasing wavelength

X-rays

Color Therapy

Color has a powerful effect on mood. It can be used to enhance or change emotions and reduce negative thoughts by encouraging positive ones to dominate. Color therapies can be used to channel energy in positive directions.

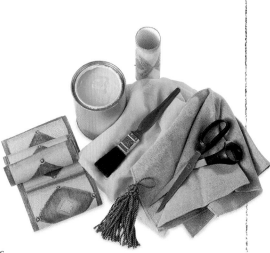

Although scientific studies of color are limited, most of us are aware of our own personal reactions to color and the effects that they can have on mood. Color therapy is an alternative treatment that uses these effects to promote healing by harnessing the radiant energy emanating from different colors. Therapists assign specific colors to various parts of the body and to specific disorders. Some therapies, including Ayurvedic medicine, use color to enhance other treatments.

One way in which color therapists work is by fixing a concentrated beam of colored light over a troubled area of the body. For example, "blue" babies have been successfully treated this way with yellow lights.

FINDING YOUR COLORS
Close your eyes and visualize different colors. Imagine yourself in a room of each color and note how you respond. Choose the colors that best suit your personal energies.

USING COLORS TO BRIGHTEN YOUR LIFE

Carefully choosing colors for your clothes and environment can help you better balance the forces within, increase your energy, and make you feel more positive. If you want to change a negative characteristic or way of thinking into a more positive one, choose a color from the list below that has attributes you would like to encourage in yourself and then surround yourself with that color. Wear the color throughout the day or use it in your environment, and positive thoughts will occur to you whenever you look at it.

COLOR ALL AROUND YOU
To improve your energy, redecorate a room in your home in a color you feel inspires energy. Alternatively, you can use the color in soft furnishings, clothes, and accessories.

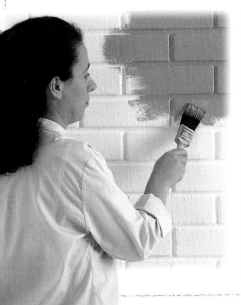

EMOTIONAL EFFECTS

Color therapists use mainly the eight colors below to encourage certain emotions and attitudes, usually by surrounding the patient with that color. White is considered to have cleansing properties.

COLOR	ATTRIBUTES
Red	Is energizing; increases vitality; helps overcome fatigue and inertia.
Orange	Promotes happiness and joy and a carefree spirit; is uplifting; helps treat depression and low energy levels.
Yellow	Promotes intellectual thought and clear thinking; improves judgment.
Green	Helps to achieve harmony and balance; cleanses and purifies the spirit.
Turquoise	Promotes calmness and strengthens immunity; helps overcome nervous tension.
Blue	Induces calm and relaxation; promotes feelings of peacefulness.
Violet	Is spiritually uplifting. Improves self-respect and esteem; provides hope.
Magenta	Encourages the breaking of stultifying habits and letting go of old emotions; promotes a sense of freedom and release.

COSMIC ENERGY FORCES: *Thunder*

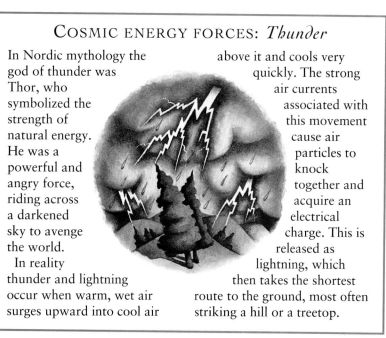

In Nordic mythology the god of thunder was Thor, who symbolized the strength of natural energy. He was a powerful and angry force, riding across a darkened sky to avenge the world.

In reality thunder and lightning occur when warm, wet air surges upward into cool air above it and cools very quickly. The strong air currents associated with this movement cause air particles to knock together and acquire an electrical charge. This is released as lightning, which then takes the shortest route to the ground, most often striking a hill or a treetop.

PROTECTING YOUR SKIN FROM THE SUN

Protecting skin against the ultraviolet (UV) rays of the sun helps to prevent burning, sunstroke, and skin cancer and is especially important for people with fair skin.

▶ *Use a protective cream or lotion with a sun-protection factor (SPF) of at least 15. It will not block UV rays but will slow them down.*

▶ *To protect your facial skin and keep your body cooler, wear a hat with a brim wide enough to shade the face.*

▶ *Move to the shade after every half hour in the sunshine.*

▶ *Cover as much skin as possible with light-colored clothing.*

---

skin disorders such as vitiligo and psoriasis. Visible blue light is employed in treating a form of jaundice that affects newborn babies.

Low-intensity lasers—when applied to damaged muscles, ligaments, tendons, and joints—will generate heat, which reduces inflammation and pain, improves the flow of blood and lymph, and stimulates tissue healing. High-intensity lasers also have many uses: cutting away scar tissue, removing abnormal cells and cancerous growths, sealing damaged blood vessels, and breaking up kidney stones and gallstones.

Most of us are aware of ultraviolet light mainly through its action on skin. UV rays activate cells in the skin to increase production of the pigment melanin, which causes the characteristic darkening that is familiar as a suntan. Overexposure to UV light, however, causes burning and skin damage.

Color therapy

Colors have long been known to have a powerful influence on mood. Those at the lower end of the visible spectrum, such as violet and blue, are considered restful and thoughtful; they are associated with peace and study and are believed to be helpful in reducing stress and anxiety. Those at the higher end, such as red, orange, and yellow, are vibrant, energetic colors associated with elation, activity, and passion.

Color therapists employ different colors for their mood-enhancing properties and for other therapeutic qualities they are thought to possess. For example, if you surround yourself with energetic colors by redecorating your rooms or wearing those hues, they may help counteract depression. Special concentrated lights can also be employed to counter specific physical problems.

X-RAY RADIATION

One of the most common forms of energy used in medical diagnosis, X-rays were discovered in 1895 by the German physicist Wilhelm Roentgen. They are part of the electromagnetic spectrum to which ultraviolet light, visible light, infrared light, and radio waves also belong.

Although invisible to the human eye, X-rays pass through softer tissues but are easily absorbed by denser tissue and bone. Because X-rays darken photographic film, they can be used to photograph bones to check for possible fractures. Images of the stomach or intestines can also be made after a patient consumes a barium meal; barium is impervious to X-rays and so outlines the organ, showing up problem areas.

Newer imaging techniques, including computed tomography (CT) scanning and positron emission tomography (PET), produce a three-dimensional view of a cross-section of the body. For a CT scan a patient is placed inside a special machine, and an X-ray unit takes hundreds of film images as it revolves around the part of the body being examined. The images are then reconstructed with a computer. To make organs stand out, a contrast dye may be used.

Radiotherapy

X-rays and other forms of radiation are used to cure disorders as well as diagnose them. This form of treatment, called radiotherapy, involves directing the X-rays at unwanted cells, such as cancerous growths, to destroy them. Early forms of radiotherapy tended to damage neighboring healthy tissue as well, but modern systems are more accurate and direct the radiation only onto the tumor. Instead of X-rays, some forms of radiotherapy involve neutron beams and substances like radioactive iodine and yttrium.

Radiotherapy is often combined with surgery and chemotherapy or drug therapy to treat cancers of the breast, larynx, skin, cervix, esophagus, and blood (leukemia). It can also be used on other conditions, such as an overactive thyroid.

THE POWER OF MAGNETISM

There is much scientific debate about the possible therapeutic effects of magnetism. It is known that an electrically generated form, called electromagnetism, plays a part in living processes, particularly nerve and muscle activity, brain function, and metabolism. In every cell there are an estimated 100,000 interactions per second that involve electromagnetism at a molecular level. Magnetism is found naturally in metals, is detectable in the earth's magnetic field, and can be produced electronically. Studies on American astronauts conducted by the National Aeronautics and Space Administration (NASA) in the 1960s showed that many were suffering from a form of space sickness caused by living for extended periods outside the earth's magnetic field, or magnetosphere. This had a serious effect on the circulation and oxygenation of their blood and was corrected only by fitting magnets to the spacecraft.

THE EARTH'S MAGNETIC FIELD

The magnetic force of the earth has a major influence on our lives. The proper functioning of astronauts' bodies is disrupted if they remain in space for extended periods.

Magnets have been used for many centuries to ease inflammatory joint disorders such as arthritis. In the late 1950s two doctors, Robert Becker and Andrew Bassett, used electromagnetic fields to treat patients with gangrene in their leg tissue. Electromagnetism proved effective in aiding tissue repair in cases in which the limb would otherwise have been at risk. Despite their success, however, the therapeutic uses of magnetism are still mostly confined to alternative health care.

Magnet therapy is based on the belief that physical disorders are mainly the result of imbalances in the electromagnetic fields generated by the body's cells. Placing magnets over the problem area is believed to have a rebalancing effect on the body and thus alleviate the disorder.

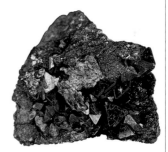

Magnetic rocks, known as bloodstones, have been mined in Africa for thousands of years and added to medicinal potions or placed on the skin to treat disease. The ancient Greeks and Chinese employed the healing properties of magnetic rocks called lodestones.

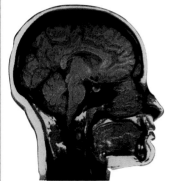

Magnetic resonance imaging (MRI) is a diagnostic technique using magnetism to build up images of the internal organs. The patient lies inside a very large electromagnet that causes atoms in the tissues to align. The atoms are then knocked out of alignment with pulses of radio waves, causing them to broadcast radio signals that can be used to build up an image. MRI can be used to examine the brain, spinal cord, heart, blood vessels, bones, and endocrine glands. It is a technique complementary to X-ray imaging.

Magnetizing water for drinking or bathing is part of traditional therapy in India. Magnetization is achieved by placing the opposite poles of two magnets on each side of a glass of water for 12 to 18 hours. To be effective, the water should be used fairly soon after the magnetizing and must not be refrigerated. The water is believed to improve health by balancing the energy forces within cells, through which it promotes vitality and strength, especially in the organs.

Electromagnetic field therapy (EMF) is a modern form of magnet therapy that is widely employed in eastern and central Europe, but less commonly in western Europe and North America. It involves the use of small portable generators that produce low-frequency, pulsating electromagnetic fields to rebalance the body. Some claim that it is useful for treating a range of conditions, including arthritis, nerve disorders, fractures, and urinary problems.

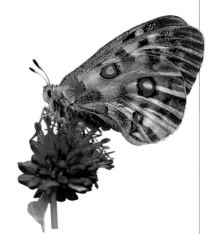

Magnetic navigation is used by many creatures for traveling. It is believed that animals such as homing pigeons and emperor butterflies can navigate vast distances by detecting and using the earth's magnetic field.

SOUND

Everybody has experienced the uplifting effects of sound through music. The therapeutic use of sound in health care is now becoming more commonplace.

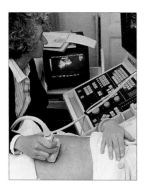

ULTRASOUND
The most common use for ultrasound imaging is to view a fetus in the mother's womb.

Sound is created by pressure, or sound, waves moving through a medium such as air or water. In the air, sound waves travel at 332 meters (1,089 feet) per second; in water, at 1,482 meters (4,863 feet) per second. When sound waves strike an object, they cause it to vibrate, or resonate.

The length of sound waves, or their frequency, varies. Only waves of a certain length resonate on the human eardrum. Sound frequencies that fall within this range are known as sonic; frequencies below this are called subsonic and above this are known as supersonic or ultrasonic.

ULTRASOUND

Ultrasonic waves are used in conventional medicine as an imaging technique called ultrasound. The basic principle behind ultrasound—echolocation—is the same as the technique that bats and dolphins use to navigate. High-frequency sound waves are directed at the part of the body to be examined, using a device called a transducer. This device also detects the echoes from internal organs and transmits them to a computer, which uses the information to create an image. The technique is most effective for examining soft tissues and fluid-filled structures, such as the heart, breasts, kidneys, liver, gallbladder, pancreas, ovaries, and testes. It is commonly used to monitor the development of an unborn baby in utero. Ultrasound is also used in physiotherapy to promote tissue growth and repair in cases of torn ligaments and strained muscles.

SOUND THERAPY

Throughout history sound has been used in different ways to treat mental and physical disorders. The simplest approach has been simply creating or listening to music. Sound employed in this way can act as a mood enhancer, relieve depression and anxiety, reduce blood pressure, and lower heartbeat.

More recently music therapy has been adopted by health professionals in North America to treat a variety of conditions. In medicine it is used to help manage pain, rehabilitate stroke and accident victims, and improve the coordination of patients who have neurological disabilities. In psychotherapy music is employed to communicate with patients who are unable to verbalize their problems, such as autistic children.

In some Eastern cultures in which sound is used to increase inner tranquillity, practitioners of sound therapy intone sounds of specific frequencies to target one of seven energy centers, or chakras, located along a straight line between the base of the spine and the crown of the head. Chakras, from the Sanskrit word for "wheel," spin faster or slower according to the energy flowing through them. To open up the energy channels and promote healing, sound is either chanted by others toward the patient or generated by an electronic device set to the correct frequency to treat the condition.

MUSIC AND DANCING
Dancing to music can not only be energizing and uplifting but also provide good exercise. A natural form of stress relief, dancing is enjoyed by every culture around the world.

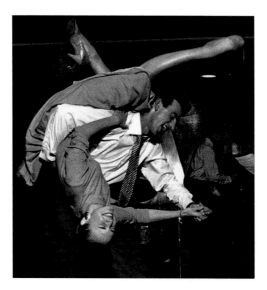

Sound Therapy

Many ancient cultures harnessed sound as a means of expressing inner emotions and used its resonance to heal the body and spirit. Sound therapy can help ease emotional problems, particularly depression and feelings connected with isolation.

Sound therapists believe that the cells of the body react to the vibrations of sound. According to their principles, the body responds well to certain tones and rhythms and unfavorably to others. The underlying theory holds that each part of the body has its own natural resonance and will vibrate in harmony with any sound of the same frequency. (This is the same principle by which a wineglass will resonate when a singer reaches a particular musical note.) Disease is thought to alter the frequency at which the affected organ or body part vibrates. Sound waves of the correct frequency vibrate the corresponding tissues so that they resonate normally again and become stronger and better able to fight disease.

Research suggests that certain musical experiences may also trigger production of endorphins, brain chemicals that are natural pain-killers. Surgeons and dentists have found that music can reduce their patients' needs for anesthesia. In cases of emotional or memory disorders, music may reach a part of the brain that is otherwise inaccessible.

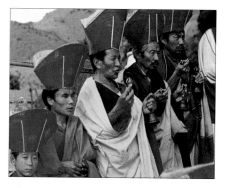

MEDITATIVE CHANTING
Many religions use the power of the human voice to inspire spiritual and emotional well-being. These Buddhist monks are chanting to gain spiritual enlightenment.

Sound is also believed to open the energy channels of the body and is used in a number of Eastern health treatments (see opposite page).

CHANTING TO RELIEVE DEPRESSION

Chanting is an ancient tradition used by many cultures to induce a spiritual, meditative, or uplifting mood. In Eastern cultures chanting is used to increase spiritual awareness and inner tranquillity. Chanting also plays a part in many Western traditions. Most religious ceremonies rely on voice to recite prayers and sing hymns in praise of nature and God, intoning the spiritual message of the ceremony.

The traditional Hindu mantra, *om*, believed to be a universal sound, consists of three parts—*aah* (which vibrates in your navel), *oo* (which vibrates in your heart), and *m* (which vibrates in your temple).

Sit comfortably and make sure you can breathe easily and deeply.

1 *Sit somewhere quiet where you can be peaceful. Relax your body so that your diaphragm moves freely. Dim the lights in the room if this helps you to concentrate. Clear your mind and breathe deeply for a few moments.*

2 *Chant your words, quietly at first. These could be the lyrics of a song you have always found uplifting or words you have made up for yourself. They could take the form of affirmations or prayer. They must be positive. For example, you could chant something like "Every day I become stronger," or "I am at one with the world," or "Love is within and around me."*

3 *After each chant, take a deep breath before you begin the next one. You may find your voice level rising as you gain confidence.*

ANIMALS, PLANTS, AND MINERALS

The life energies within nature can be drawn upon to balance your own energies, and so can the energy from the mineral elements that form a basis for all life.

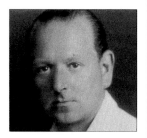

DR. EDWARD BACH
Edward Bach, a British physician, dedicated his life to working out links between nature and human health. His flower remedies, taken to relieve certain emotional states, were based on the belief that our emotions and experiences shape our physical health.

THE STRENGTH OF THE ANIMALS
Traditionally, Native Americans have used the feathers of birds of prey in headdresses and costumes to give themselves strength and protection.

The energy of plants and minerals has been used for thousands of years to promote health and vitality. The ancient Egyptians were especially interested in taking advantage of the energies of both plants and minerals, especially precious stones, which were mounted in jewelry or ornaments to preserve positive energies. According to traditional Chinese medicine, energies from herbs and stones can contribute greatly to energy balance in humans.

Native Americans have long used feathers, particularly from birds of prey, to partake of the birds' energies. The skins and furs of animals—particularly powerful species—have also been used for this purpose so that the wearer can take on the characteristic strength of, say, a bear or a buffalo. Many other cultures around the world, notably the peoples of West Africa, have used the teeth and bones from various animals for their energizing qualities.

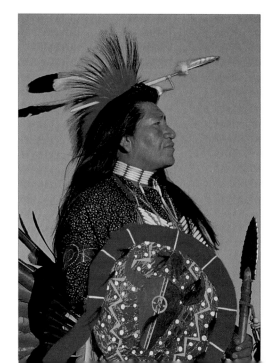

HOMEOPATHY

Homeopathic medicine puts great store in the concept of an energy, or "vital force," that exists in plants, minerals, and other natural substances. In homeopathy the plant essences are extracted in a water-ethanol medium. The mixture is diluted and shaken repeatedly in a process called succession, which is believed to transfer the vital force of the ingredients to the water.

Homeopathic remedies are based on the principle of "like cures like." Substances that in large doses produce symptoms that mimic those of a particular disease will, in small amounts, actually cure the illness. The therapy was prompted by the discovery that cinchona bark, from which the antimalarial drug quinine is extracted, itself produces malaria-like symptoms, such as fever.

The active ingredients in homeopathic remedies are so dilute that no trace of the original ingredient can be detected. Yet numerous studies have shown that homeopathic remedies can be highly beneficial in alleviating a wide range of illnesses. Some practitioners believe that this is because the process of succession transfers the ingredient's vital force to the water's molecular structure. While there are many theories, no clear and coherent explanation of how homeopathy works has yet been proposed.

FLOWER REMEDIES

Extracts of flowers and other plants have been used for thousands of years to treat illnesses, but their active ingredients can also be diluted, like homeopathic remedies, in order to enhance their vital force. The best-known exponent of the healing powers of flowers was Edward Bach, a practicing doctor and homeopath in the early 20th century. Bach devised a simple treatment system based on 38 flower remedies. He believed that the essence of the flower could be extracted by allowing it to float on clear spring water in sunlight for a few hours.

Flower remedies are used mainly for alleviating psychological disorders, such as mental trauma, stress, and depression. According to Bach, his flower remedies contain a life force that vibrates at a higher level than mere flesh and blood.

MINERALS

Minerals have been used for many years as sources of decoration, and special forces have been attributed to some. Until the last centur, folk doctors applied gold leaf to wounds in order to speed healing, although their success was questionable. Other metals reputedly endowed with special forces include silver and copper.

CRYSTALS

Because of their precise structure, crystals resonate at a constant rate, which is the reason quartz crystals are used in watches to keep accurate time. When quartz crystals are put in an electromagnetic field, they vibrate at a high frequency, thus producing ultrasonic sounds. This is the principle behind ultrasound scanners. By bouncing these sounds off internal organs in the body they can be used to investigate medical disorders.

Crystal therapy

The precise structures of crystals, often in arrangements of cubes or octahedrons (eight-sided figures), have long fascinated alternative therapists. People who use crystals as part of their healing methods believe that certain stones contain powerful energy forces that can help heal physical, mental, emotional, and spiritual ills by correcting imbalances in the vibration patterns of the body's tissues.

Sometimes crystals on a pendulum are used to aid in diagnosis. The therapist suspends a crystal over the area of the body being investigated and by its movements locates the underlying cause. To treat a condition, a crystal may be placed next to the body for a while, or individuals may be told to wear the crystal or carry it around with them. Some people sew small pockets inside their garments in which to carry crystals.

Crystal-essence therapy involves the use of purified water that has been energized through contact with crystals in bright sunlight. The individual places a few drops of the liquid remedy under the tongue at certain times of the day.

In electrocrystal therapy electricity is used to increase the resonance of crystals. The crystals are placed in a saline-filled glass tube and sealed. The tube is then placed on the body and electrically stimulated at a pulse rate that matches the natural resonance of the part of the body being treated.

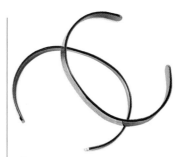

COPPER BRACELETS FOR ARTHRITIS Research carried out in Australia in the early 1980s found that the copper in a bracelet can penetrate skin and act as an anti-inflammatory agent on arthritis and rheumatism.

THE ENERGY OF STONES

With their regular shapes and smooth surfaces, crystals are created by the strong electromagnetic attraction of one atom to others of the same kind. Some therapists see this as evidence of great energy and healing power. A number of semiprecious stones are associated with particular powers. Some people wear or carry crystals; others keep them in their homes.

HEALING STONES? Crystal therapy associates each crystal with a different physical, mental, or spiritual attribute, some examples of which are shown here. They may be used individually or in combination.

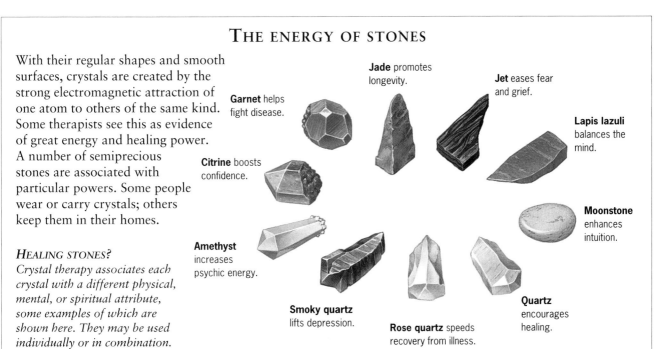

Jade promotes longevity.

Jet eases fear and grief.

Garnet helps fight disease.

Lapis lazuli balances the mind.

Citrine boosts confidence.

Moonstone enhances intuition.

Amethyst increases psychic energy.

Smoky quartz lifts depression.

Rose quartz speeds recovery from illness.

Quartz encourages healing.

THE FIVE ENERGIES

Ayurveda and traditional Chinese medicine share a belief in five principal forces of energy that govern the world around us, as well as our own physical, mental, and psychological health.

THE FIVE ELEMENTS AND YOUR BODY

In Chinese medicine each of the five elements is believed to be connected to a yin and a yang part of the body (see opposite page). If you have an imbalance in your elements, it may manifest itself physically in the related region.

▶ *Wood has the liver as the yin organ and the gallbladder as the yang.*

▶ *Fire's yin organ is the heart, and its yang is the small intestine.*

▶ *Earth can be found in the spleen (yin) and the stomach (yang).*

▶ *Metal has the lungs as its yin organ and the large intestine as its yang.*

▶ *Water's yin organ is the kidney, and the yang is the bladder.*

SEASONS AND ENERGY
According to traditional Chinese medicine, your energy levels are strongly affected by the dominant energy force of the season. For example, spring is characterized by young yang energy and the element wood. This energy force can tend toward excess and aggression, and so some therapists recommend yin foods to achieve balance (see page 75).

Many people are aware of the influence of the seasons and weather on their moods and energy levels. For some, a change in temperature or humidity may bring about illness or pain or aggravate an existing condition such as asthma. However, in Ayurveda and traditional Chinese medicine, five fundamental energy forces of nature are seen as directing our health and well-being. Good health involves maintaining a proper balance of these five basic energies.

AYURVEDIC MEDICINE
Ayurvedic medicine, which originated in India over 5,000 years ago, is based on an understanding of *prana*, the natural energy, or life force. According to Ayurvedic teaching, nature and all matter, people included, are made up of five elements: earth, water, fire, air, and ether (space). In different combinations, these elements make up the three principles, or tridoshas—*vata, kapha,* and *pita*—that govern all things.

The principle of the three doshas is at the heart of Ayurveda (see page 50). Each is made up of combinations of two of the five elements. Vata, which represents winter, combines ether and air and controls movement. Kapha, representing spring, combines water and earth. It is responsible for growth and structure, the solid, unmoving factor. Pita, signifying summer, combines fire and water and is responsible for metabolism.

As people are considered to be a microcosm of the natural world, they, too, are defined by one or more of the tridoshas and their relevant elements. Ayurvedic treatments aim to balance the tridoshas, bringing all the elements into harmony and helping a person to understand his or her strengths and weaknesses.

THE FIVE ELEMENT THEORY
The principles of Ayurveda eventually spread to China, where they were modified and, over time, developed into the principles of traditional Chinese medicine. The equivalent to prana is chi (also written qi), which means "breath" or "spirit." It is the life force or vital energy found in all living things and forms the five elements—fire, air, wood, metal, and earth.

The basis of this belief is that each person should have a balance of the five elements; if one is dominant or submissive, it should be balanced by using an opposing one to control or nourish the problem area. Energy problems are investigated and diagnosed by examining the body, mental attitude, and emotions. Commonly a patient has a specific condition that needs treatment, such as a stomach problem, which would be identified as an earth disorder. The treatment would encourage strength and balance of the earth energy by stifling the controlling force and encouraging the nourishing force.

Practitioners treat imbalances with a combination of remedies, including dietary measures, lifestyle changes, herbalism, massage (Tuina), exercises (*chi kung*), and acupuncture. A psychological element helps with

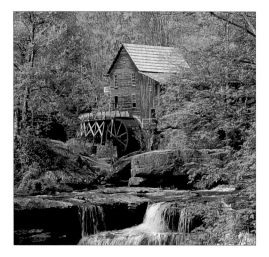

THE FIVE ELEMENTS

This theory holds that each person is created from a mixture of five elements, or energies, with one predominating; a balance of all five results in good health and energy. Sometimes people have imbalances that affect their physical and psychological makeup. Once a problem is identified by matching the symptoms and element, the problem element is then controlled or strengthened by observing and treating other elements through herbal therapy, acupuncture, changes in diet and mental attitude, and exercises. You can find out what your astrological element is from the table on page 52.

Fire
stands for reason and expression; it nourishes earth. Fire people are forceful, influential, and capable but have a tendency to be intolerant, aggressive, and judgmental. Those lacking in fire are unmotivated.

Wood
stands for steadfastness and benevolence; it nourishes fire. Those with wood predominating are like sturdy trees, resilient and sheltering, but they cannot bend to new ideas. A person lacking in wood is easily influenced.

Earth
stands for honesty and loyalty; it nourishes metal. Those with earth predominating are earnest, self-sacrificing, and generous, but they can be procrastinators, avoiding the realities of life. People with little earth tend to be self-centered.

Controls

Water
nourishes wood and is divided into two phases: moving and still. Moving water represents drive and success. Still water stands for insight, reflection, and intelligence. A person lacking in water is narrow-minded.

Metal
stands for righteousness; it nourishes water. Metal people are prone to be talkative, argumentative, confident, and opinionated. A person lacking in metal can be quiet, isolated, and aloof.

both diagnosis and treatment and can also be used for predictions, especially in combination with Chinese astrology. The holistic approach of traditional Chinese medicine stresses the direct links between the body and personality and behavior. A change in lifestyle and attitude is often considered equally as important as physical treatments to restore health and vitality.

Traditional Chinese practitioners believe that there are other powerful forces in nature, as well as chi and the five elements. The most important of these are yin and yang, which are seen as opposing yet complementary poles, forces, or principles. Yin is the cool, passive, feminine force, while yang is the warm, active, masculine force. Yin and yang exist in all things in different proportions but maintain a state of equilibrium unless malign forces upset this balance. An imbalance in yin and yang causes disharmony in nature and illness in people. Chinese medicine is aimed at restoring and maintaining the balance between the two forces.

CHINESE ASTROLOGY AND THE FIVE ELEMENTS

Traditional Chinese philosophy suggests that each year is represented by an animal and an element and that these will dictate *continued on page 52*

DID YOU KNOW?

Western astrology and the study of star signs originated in India and are based on a traditional reading of the stars and planets to perceive the changes and imbalances in universal forces. Astrology is founded on a system of 12 signs, each dependent on the changing arrangements of the stars and planets throughout the year. Every sign has a ruling element, although Western astrology recognizes only four elements: earth, air, water, and fire. These are believed to affect the personality and health of each individual in a fashion similar to the Ayurvedic elements and the Chinese elements.

How it works

The following example illustrates how the five element theory works in practice. If you have a kidney problem, you may have a water disorder. Since earth controls water, your problem may be due to an overactive soil element, possibly originating in the spleen or stomach. It would be treated by nourishing water with metal foods and emotions. You may also need to consider the psychological aspects of the problem: are you anxious about anything? What do you have to fear?

Ayurveda Practitioner

The principle of energy balancing has a central role in Ayurvedic medicine. The therapy takes a holistic approach to ailments and examines how diet, exercise, and emotions work together to influence health and energy levels.

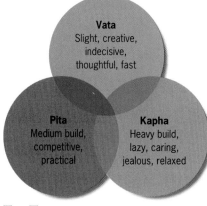

THE TRIDOSHA
Ayurvedic tradition holds that each person is a mixture of three characters, or doshas, that have different physical and emotional natures, and one dosha predominates. If you have a health problem, you are assessed for which dosha is out of balance, and this forms the basis of treatment.

Ayurveda, the traditional and all-encompassing medical system of India, derives its name from the Sanskrit for "life" (*ayur*) and "knowledge" (*veda*). The practice is holistic, aiming to treat imbalances of mind, body, and spirit to promote good health and combat illness. It is widely used in India alongside orthodox medicine and is steadily gaining interest in the West, especially with widespread popularity of one of its noted practitioners, Deepak Chopra.

How does Ayurvedic medicine work?
Ayurvedic medicine is based on the concept of prana (energy). It is believed that this energy is forever fluctuating, changing from negative to positive and back again, and controls our physical, emotional, mental, and spiritual health. The aim of Ayurvedic practice is to balance or promote more positive energy in all four of these areas to allow patients to achieve their full potential in life.

According to Ayurvedic philosophy, each person is born with a particular ratio of the three doshas—vata, pita, and kapha—with one predominating. Your dominant dosha determines your shape, constitution, coloring, personality, and temperament, as well as the types of illness you might be susceptible to. It also determines how you will be treated by an ayurvedic practitioner.

How are practitioners qualified?
In India practitioners undergo five years of training in an Ayurdevic medical school and a year of internship. In Canada and the United States this training is abbreviated to several months at an Ayurvedic institute. However, to practice Ayurvedic medicine, a person must also have a degree in traditional medicine or osteopathy. Otherwise, only consultation work is permitted.

What happens during a session?
Ayurvedic practitioners believe that the way an individual reacts to the world and is influenced by it are important factors in health. They accept that not all remedies work in the same way for everyone. The skill of the practitioner is to identify and prescribe treatment that will work for the individual. To achieve this,

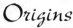

Origins
Ayurveda originated in India some 5,000 years ago and is probably the oldest medical system in the world. According to tradition, 52 wise and holy men went to the Himalayas, as they believed the mountains were close to universal forces. There they meditated on how they could eradicate illness from the world. Their meditations, which they thought were divinely inspired, led them to devise systems to promote good health. They wrote them down in the *Charaka Samhita*, regarded as a sacred text.

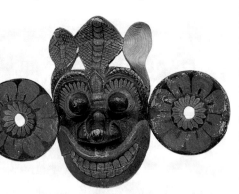

HEALING MASK
Masks are traditionally used to ward off the demons that upset the balance of the tridosha. This mask represents Garayaka, the demon of purification, and is worn to exorcize the evil spirit. It is from Sri Lanka and is dated between 1771 and 1910.

the Ayurvedic doctor aims to find out as much as possible about each patient. This will include seeking details not only about you, but also your parents and grandparents, from whom you inherited characteristics.

You will be questioned about your diet and lifestyle, perhaps even your dreams. Finally, your symptoms will be investigated. This will include further questioning, followed by a physical examination of the eyes, nose, tongue, nails, feet, skin, and hair, and the taking of pulses in many parts of the body; this last is an important diagnostic method.

What type of treatment is given?

Treatment is given not just for the condition but also to improve your whole life. Diet and lifestyle changes may be advised, as well as medication. First, however, the body must be cleansed of wastes. This could involve massage with oils to promote internal equilibrium, followed by sweat therapy to eliminate wastes from the body. Panchakarma, internal detoxification to remove toxins, involves emetics, fasting, and steam inhalations.

Sometimes rejuvenation therapy (Rasayana) is necessary for a long-term illness. This aims to boost the immune system and mental faculties. Yoga, meditation, and counseling may also be advised.

Natural herbal remedies are often prescribed. These have been in use within Ayurvedic practice for thousands of years, but many are also known in the West. The Indian and Sri Lankan governments fund ongoing research in Ayurvedic medicine, and drug companies in the West are also doing research. The Ayurvedic medical authorities keep updated databases on the results of such research and this can be referred to by qualified practitioners.

Can Ayurvedic medicine improve energy levels?

In Ayurvedic medicine, marma therapy is used to influence body functions. It works like acupressure,

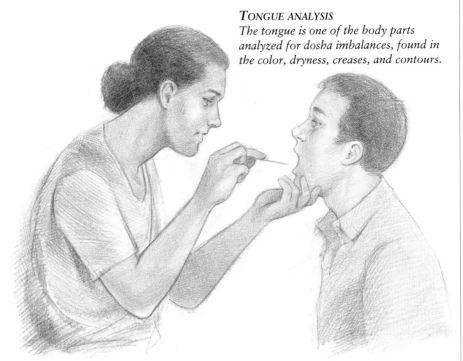

TONGUE ANALYSIS
The tongue is one of the body parts analyzed for dosha imbalances, found in the color, dryness, creases, and contours.

relating specific disorders to points on the body. The point that relates to lack of energy is situated at the top of the head; this point is also associated with headaches and memory problems. Applying gentle pressure to the point energizes it or depresses it, depending on which is required. However, a practitioner will also advise on an energizing diet specific to your dosha type and your lifestyle to further promote energy.

What can Ayurvedic medicine treat?

Ayurvedic medicine works as a complement to orthodox medicine, supporting rather than replacing it; a range of disorders can be treated. However, it is particularly suitable for conditions such as irritable bowel syndrome, chronic fatigue syndrome, flu, depression, insomnia, anxiety, asthma, joint conditions such as arthritis, and a wide range of skin conditions like eczema and dermatitis.

WHAT YOU CAN DO AT HOME

Most Ayurvedic medicine must be prescribed by a practitioner, but given here are simple home remedies that can relieve minor illnesses.

Headaches and sinus problems

Boil 60 milliliters (¼ cup) coriander seeds in water for 10 minutes, transfer to a bowl, and then inhale the steam to clear the nasal passages.

Colds

Gently brown 60 milliliters (¼ cup) coriander seeds in a pan, add 1 liter (1 quart) water and 4 slices fresh ginger, and boil until volume is reduced by half; strain and drink.

Indigestion

Slice some fresh ginger and chew it thoroughly to extract the juice. Swallow the juice and discard the chewed pulp.

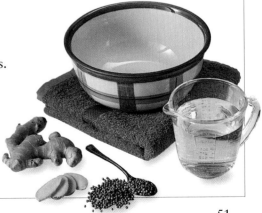

the occurrences during that year and the nature of the people born in that year. Your animal and your element are used to determine your strengths and weaknesses and predict your destiny. They are frequently used to explain relationships and compatibility with friends and family. The diagram on page 49 describes the principal characteristics of each element and shows how it relates to the others, all of them interlinking and working as a whole system.

The Chinese take their astrology very seriously, and many follow the predictions with great fervor. The compatibility of marriage partnerships is often determined according to astrological links. Couples frequently plan their children to fall within certain years—the most popular being the year of the Dragon, with the year of the Snake coming in a close second. Some years are also avoided if possible; traditionally, female babies born in the year of the Fire Horse (which occurs once every 60 years) were killed at birth because it was felt that they were too rebellious and uncontrollable to suit the traditional female temperament.

THE FIVE ELEMENTS AND CHINESE ASTROLOGY

Your astrological animal and element are indicated by the year in which you were born. If, however, you were born in January (before the Chinese new year), you are considered part of the previous year. The characteristics of the astrological animals are given in the table below. For a description of your element, see the diagram on page 49. The animal describes your character tendencies, whereas the element explains your deeper emotional status and the relationships with those around you. The animal and element of the current year are used for predictions of future events and how you may be put out of balance by changing energy forces. Advice often focuses on diet and behavioral changes to rebalance your energies and avoid misfortune.

ELEMENT	METAL	WATER	W00D	FIRE	EARTH	CHARACTERISTICS
Rat	1900 1960	1912 1972	1924 1984	1936 1996	1948 2008	Restless, aggressive, charming, successful, discontented, expressive, perfectionist, stubborn, adamant
Ox	1901 1961	1913 1973	1925 1985	1937 1997	1949 2009	Diligent, patient, observant, good memory, dogmatic, hard-working, practical, strong-willed
Tiger	1950 2010	1902 1962	1914 1974	1926 1986	1938 1998	Powerful, leader, daring, magnetic, confident, authoritative, good fighter, warm-hearted, dominating, egotistical
Rabbit	1951 2011	1903 1963	1915 1975	1927 1987	1939 1999	Delicate, kind, loving, popular, cool, conservative, insecure, pessimistic, well-dressed, lovable, peaceful, sensitive, lucky
Dragon	1940 2000	1952 2012	1904 1964	1916 1976	1928 1988	Noble, masterful, powerful, perfectionist, influential, dynamic, inflexible, lucky, idealist, stubborn, forceful
Snake	1941 2001	1953 2013	1905 1965	1917 1977	1929 1989	Diplomatic, charming, popular, deep-thinking, intellectual, intuitive, perceptive, thoughtful, inspired, charismatic, ostentatious
Horse	1930 1990	1942 2002	1954 2014	1906 1966	1918 1978	Energetic, hot-blooded, rebellious, impatient, quick-witted, cunning, selfish, productive, sociable, capable, independent
Goat	1931 1991	1943 2003	1955 2015	1907 2067	1919 1979	Gentle, elegant, creative, charming, dreamers, lazy, insecure, pessimistic, relaxed, self-centered, lovable
Monkey	1920 1980	1932 2092	1944 2004	1956 2016	1908 1968	Merry, fun, loving, cheerful, generous, deceptive, clever, diplomatic, creative, sociable, carefree, energetic
Rooster	1921 1981	1933 2093	1945 2005	1957 2017	1909 1969	Enthusiastic, observant, accurate, attention-seeking, cautious, perceptive, analyzing, resourceful, practical
Dog	1910 1970	1922 1982	1934 1994	1946 2006	1958 2018	Dutiful, honest, faithful, sincere, honorable, loyal, caring, defensive, judgmental, loving, jealous, amicable
Pig	1911 1971	1923 1983	1935 1995	1947 2007	1959 2019	Chivalrous, sincere, tolerant, honorable, admirable, loving, generous, companionable, obliging, thoughtful, considerate

CHAPTER 3

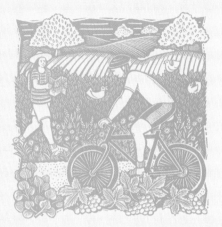

ENERGY DRAINERS

Many lifestyle factors can have a significant influence on your energy levels. Increasing your awareness of how you are affected by your working and living environments, your emotional state, your dietary habits, even your use of common drugs such as caffeine or aspirin, can help you to maximize your energy and improve your health.

SLEEP AND ENERGY

The duration and quality of sleep have a profound effect on daytime performance, as well as on health, a sense of well-being, and, in fact, the whole quality of life.

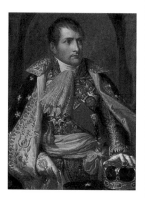

SLEEPING PATTERNS
Napoleon regularly slept for fewer than five hours each night. However, he slept for 36 hours after his defeat in the Battle of Aspern in 1809—the first battle that the French emperor lost after 17 successive triumphs.

Sleep plays an essential part in the body's daily routine. It allows tired muscles to rest, depleted energy levels to be restored, and tissues to repair themselves. Sleep also allows the conscious mind to rest and recuperate and enables the unconscious mind to store the skills and knowledge acquired during the day. The young of all species sleep longer than adults, and the amount of sleep that individuals need diminishes with age, suggesting that sleep may be particularly important for growth, development, and learning.

REVITALIZING YOUR BODY

As you drift off to sleep, your muscles become more relaxed, your heartbeat and breathing rate slow down, blood pressure drops, and temperature falls. The digestive system remains active, although your metabolic rate decreases by about 20 percent. Some senses, such as hearing, continue to monitor any changes in your surroundings, but the deeper the sleep, the less responsive the brain becomes to external stimuli. All these processes are important for proper rest and recuperation of the body and mind, encouraging renewal of energy and alertness during waking hours.

On average, adults need about eight hours of sleep, although this figure drops to about four to six hours in old age. Sleep requirements vary from person to person and from day to day, however, depending on the individual's sex, activity levels, and environment, as well as genetic and general health factors. Many people need more or less than the average amount as a matter of course or on particular days of the week.

Too little sleep is a common problem affecting daytime energy levels, as well as physical and psychological well-being. Generally, a longer sleep provides periods of deeper sleep, allowing the body to recuperate more completely. Poor, unrefreshing sleep is considered by some doctors to be a significant factor in myalgic encephalomyelitis (ME), or chronic fatigue syndrome (CFS), an increasingly common condition.

Energy levels can also be affected by too much sleep. It has been found that excessive sleep can lead to fatigue, lack of motivation, a loss of alertness, and an inability to make decisions. Many people with CFS find that regularly sleeping for more than 11 hours a day can worsen their symptoms. In these cases restricting sleep to an average of eight to nine hours may help to reduce fatigue.

Having an irregular sleep pattern can also lead to fatigue and difficulty concentrating. Changes in sleep patterns between weekdays and weekends is thought by sleep-disorder specialists to contribute to the general feeling of lethargy known as the "Monday morning feeling." Sleep and disease are intricately related, and excessive drowsiness may

SLEEP AND AGE

Babies sleep the most, although rarely for long periods at a time. At about six months, they start to develop a normal day/night pattern. As people grow older, they need less sleep but they also have more problems with sleeplessness.

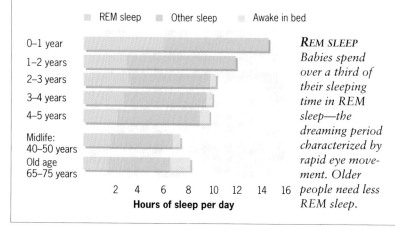

| | REM sleep | Other sleep | Awake in bed |

0–1 year
1–2 years
2–3 years
3–4 years
4–5 years
Midlife: 40–50 years
Old age 65–75 years

2 4 6 8 10 12 14 16
Hours of sleep per day

REM SLEEP
Babies spend over a third of their sleeping time in REM sleep—the dreaming period characterized by rapid eye movement. Older people need less REM sleep.

be a symptom of a serious condition, for example, a brain disorder, head injury, hormonal problem, or liver failure.

SLEEP DISORDERS

Sleep apnea, characterized by heavy snoring and periods during which the person stops breathing repeatedly for anywhere from 10 seconds to 2 or 3 minutes, is a fairly common disorder that often goes undetected. The most common type, obstructive sleep apnea, is caused by an obstruction to the passage of air from enlarged tonsils or adenoids or over-relaxation of the muscles in the soft palate.

The condition mainly affects overweight middle-aged men, although it can occur at any age and in either sex. (In adults with the disorder, there is an increased risk of sudden death from a heart attack; in infants, a risk of sudden infant death syndrome.) Another type of sleep apnea is caused by a malfunction of the brain's respiratory center. The airway is open but the respiratory structures do not receive the correct messages from the brain.

INSOMNIA

Insomnia is the term used to describe such sleep problems as difficulty in falling asleep, repeated waking, and early waking before the sleep cycle is complete. It is a common complaint, experienced by around 40 percent of adults at some time in their lives. Insufficient or disturbed sleep commonly leads to aching and tired muscles and feelings of lethargy the following day. It can be caused by a number of factors, including pain or general discomfort, stress, noise, or hormonal changes, such as those that occur during pregnancy. Most cases of insomnia are temporary and do not pose a significant threat to health. However, long-term insomnia can seriously affect the sufferer's quality of life, and professional medical help should be sought. In some cases sleeping pills may provide temporary relief, but medication seldom provides a satisfactory solution, as it can interfere with sleep patterns and lead to drug tolerance, requiring progressively larger doses to achieve the same effect.

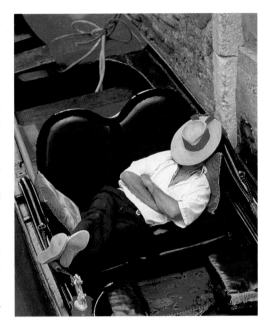

Mild cases of sleep apnea can be alleviated usually with remedies for snoring (see pages 58–59). In more severe cases surgery may be necessary. Also, a positive-airflow machine, which blows air into the nose, can help keep the upper airways open. Alcohol and sleeping pills can aggravate the condition.

HYPERSOMNIA AND NARCOLEPSY

Hypersomnia, or excessive sleep, can cause daytime drowsiness. This is a recognized medical problem; hypersomniacs are lacking in energy and enthusiasm and run the risk of becoming caffeine or amphetamine addicts to keep themselves awake.

In most women there may be minor sleep changes with the menstrual cycle and during pregnancy. Periodic hypersomnia has been linked to menstruation since 1943, when the first case was reported in a 14-year-old girl. She slept deeply for four or five days, beginning on the fourth day of her menstrual cycle; when awake, the girl ate excessively. A number of similar examples of menstrual hypersomnolence have since been reported, though not all have featured overeating. Hypersomnia during menstruation may cease when ovulation is stopped by oral contraceptive pills.

Certain medications and excessive intake of alcohol can also cause hypersomnia and lethargy. This is because stimulants alter the brain's normal sleep patterns, leading to disturbed sleep. In people who already suffer a sleep disorder, excessive intake of alcohol and drugs can exacerbate the problem.

SIESTA TIME
In warm climates many workers take an afternoon rest, or siesta, every day. A siesta can last from 20 minutes to 2 hours and is normally taken after a long lunch—the main meal of the day. It enables people to relax while they digest their meal and also allows them to rest rather than work during the hottest time of the day. Businesses and shops reopen later in the day and usually stay open until late evening.

TIPS ON AVOIDING INSOMNIA

Here are techniques that can help combat insomnia:

▶ *Develop a regular bedtime routine.*

▶ *No matter how tired you feel, don't lie in bed later than normal in the morning.*

▶ *Avoid a heavy meal and excess alcohol too late in the evening.*

▶ *Have a warm caffeine-free drink and toast or crackers before bed.*

▶ *Sprinkle a few drops of lavender oil on your pillow.*

▶ *Take a warm bath with relaxing aromatherapy oils.*

▶ *Exercise vigorously at least three times a week.*

▶ *Learn a relaxation technique, such as deep breathing, that you can do at bedtime.*

▶ *Don't lie in bed worrying; if you can't sleep, get up and do something else until you feel sleepier.*

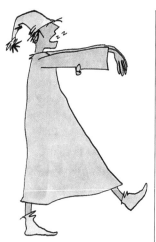

MOBILE SLEEPER
Sleepwalking can be a frightening experience. Although it is not dangerous to wake a sleepwalker, it is sensible to guide him or her gently back to bed while still sleeping.

In an extreme but rare form of persistent daytime drowsiness called narcolepsy, a person falls asleep repeatedly throughout the day. Frequency of attacks is unrelated to the amount of sleep received. Sufferers may also experience sudden muscle collapse, called cataplexy, as well as hallucinations and dreams while awake. The disorder, which can be highly disruptive to a person's life, is usually treated with a stimulant such as ephedrine.

OTHER SLEEP DISORDERS

Sleepwalking, or somnambulism, occurs when a sleeping person gets out of bed and moves around without waking. Up to 25 percent of people experience this at least once in their lives, usually in childhood. It most often affects children between ages 5 and 10 and is usually outgrown by the age of 15. Another disorder, night terrors, occurs when a person, normally a young child, awakens from a deep sleep with a sense of great fear, pounding pulse, and labored breathing. Most people grow out of these traumatic experiences, and those who reach adulthood and are still having night terrors are advised to seek help to find the underlying cause of the problem.

JET LAG

Long-distance air travel that crosses several time zones causes people to change their normal sleep patterns. Travelers suddenly have to fit in with meal and sleep times of a different time zone while their internal body clock is still functioning in the time pattern of the region they have just left. In most people the result is jet lag: sleepiness and fatigue during the waking period and insomnia during the sleep period. The severity of the condition increases according to the number of time zones crossed. Regular travelers often find that westbound flights are less disruptive than eastbound flights because of the westward movement of the sun.

Both sleepwalking and night terrors differ from dreams or nightmares in that they occur during deep, dreamless sleep periods and not during the REM phase. The causes are unknown, but they are more common

SLEEP PATTERNS

As you fall asleep, you pass through various stages of sleep, which are categorized according to the level of brain activity. The lightest sleep occurs just after you have fallen asleep, and dreaming is done during this period, known as the rapid eye movement (REM) stage because of the visible eye movements that take place as you dream. The next four stages take you to progressively deeper sleep until you reach the deepest level, stage 4. During a normal sleep period, you pass from stage 1 to stage 4 and back again several times without waking up. As you go through the lighter sleep stages, you pass through REM sleep, possibly a

few times a night, on average. The longer you sleep, the shorter will be the periods of deep sleep and the longer the lighter, REM periods, which is the reason people often wake up while still dreaming.

SLEEP CHART
When you go to sleep at night, your body gradually goes into deep sleep, progressing through REM sleep (colored yellow) and the four stages. You may remain in deep sleep for a while before returning to light sleep. The graph below shows the progression of a normal night's sleep for an average sleeper over a seven-hour period.

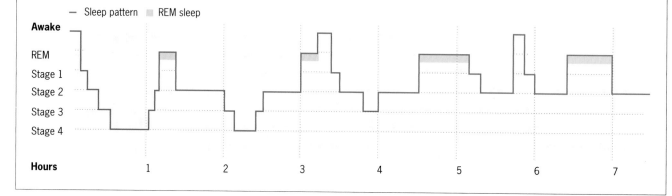

during times of anxiety and stress and tend to run in families. If the condition is persistent, you should seek professional help.

ALTERED SLEEP PATTERNS

In some situations, usually work related, people have to adapt to unnatural sleep patterns. A common example is working in shifts, which has long been an accepted pattern of working life for many people. It has been estimated that up to a third of male workers and a fifth of female workers do some form of rotation in their jobs.

In such occupations as security and factory work, people may do continual night shifts. This requires a major adjustment to the normal sleep cycle, as it involves sleeping during the day, when the body is naturally at its most active, and working at night, when the body would normally be at rest.

THE EFFECTS OF DREAMING

On average, dreaming occurs four or five times during the night, in sessions lasting 5 to 20 minutes. It is thought that deprivation of dream sleep can lead to learning problems in children and psychological difficulties in adults. People who do not get enough dream sleep often suffer reduced alertness and vitality. In experiments people who

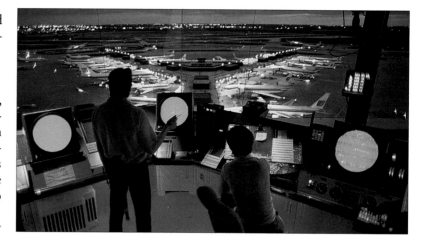

have been deprived of dream sleep become irritable, lose concentration, and may even hallucinate. Subsequent sleep periods contain a higher than normal proportion of dream sleep to enable them to catch up. A lack of dream sleep can also occur as a result of taking sleeping pills or drugs; they can keep the mind in a state of deep sleep and prevent proper REM dream stages, which are necessary for the mind to sort out problems and deal with emotions.

Dream periods become longer and more frequent according to the length of time that is spent asleep. Babies and young children, who spend much more time sleeping than adults do, have longer periods of dream sleep, and this pattern has been linked to mental development and the promotion of brain activity. Although the actual purpose of dreams has never been fully understood, many psychologists believe that the subconscious—the instinctive portion of the mind that is hidden from the conscious, rational part—expresses itself through dreams, helping individuals to work through complex emotional and psychological problems. A number of therapies incorporate dream analysis to help uncover a person's problems and frustrations.

Some people remember their dreams very vividly, while others rarely realize that they have been dreaming. Most people, however, experience nightmares at some point during their lives, when they are awakened by an unpleasant dream with a powerful emotional content of anxiety, terror, or dread of death. Nightmares occur most often in childhood, when the periods of REM sleep are longer and more frequent. As people age, they become more adapted to their experiences and need to dream less.

ALCOHOL AND SLEEP

Alcohol can severely disrupt the quality of sleep. Research has shown that going to bed after drinking sends you quickly into a deep sleep, but when the sedating effect of the alcohol wears off, you may wake up and find it difficult to get to sleep again.

Small doses of alcohol can help you relax, but more than a couple of glasses of wine or beer can lead to sleeping problems. A typical result is deep sleep for three to four hours, followed by recurrent waking with sweating, headaches, and intense dreams or nightmares. Long-term sleeping problems due to alcoholism have a marked effect on energy levels and mental well-being. In heavy drinkers sudden abstinence can also cause insomnia. For sound sleep it is best to drink alcohol moderately or not at all.

WORKING SHIFTS
Up to 80 percent of people who work in shifts suffer serious sleep-related disorders, typically drowsiness and lethargy at work and insomnia at home. There is little doubt that people function best in the normal sleeping/waking cycle, and that in all shift situations, concentration and decision-making, and hence performance, tend to suffer.

Snoring

Snoring affects not only the people who do it but also those around them, especially their partners, who may be prevented from getting a good night's sleep. The inevitable result is tiredness, loss of concentration and vitality, and irritability.

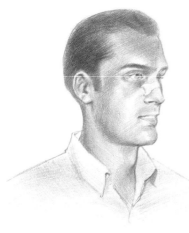

DEVICES THAT STOP SNORING
A lightweight nose plaster pulls open the nasal passages, allowing you to breathe more easily through your upper nose. Available from drugstores and supermarkets, they are relatively inexpensive.

Snoring occurs when the tissues inside the nose and throat partially block the windpipe, preventing easy breathing. Sleep apnea, a more serious snoring condition, occurs when the tissues become flabby and cause breathing to stop completely for several seconds, sometimes even a couple of minutes, before the brain triggers a gasping or snoring response to restore breathing. This response usually awakens the sleeper slightly, which opens the airways once again and the whole process

starts over. Getting a good night's sleep is difficult because of these persistent disruptions, and sufferers inevitably find themselves feeling tired and lacking in energy.

Snoring is more likely to affect anyone over the age of 30 because muscle tone is lost with increasing age. It is also more prevalent in people who are overweight, particularly middle-aged men. Other conditions can also contribute to snoring, such as a tumor or cyst in the airway.

LIVING WITH A SNORING PROBLEM

There are a number of actions you can take to help reduce or relieve snoring. Making a few changes in lifestyle and becoming more health conscious will help most snorers, although more serious cases usually require more drastic measures. Corrective surgery can be done to remove or "tuck" the tissue that is causing the problem, but doctors generally resort to this procedure only if the condition is so severe it has become dangerous.

DON'T STRAIN YOURSELF
Going to bed when overtired or absolutely exhausted can compound a snoring problem by relaxing your muscles and tissues and allowing them to block your airways. Avoid fatigue by taking brief rests during the day and try go to bed at a reasonable time every night.

▶ *If you are overweight, slimming down usually decreases snoring dramatically. A study in the United States has found that a 10 to 25 percent drop in weight significantly improves snoring problems and apnea. This is because the excess weight puts pressure on the tissues and encourages sagging.*

▶ *Give up cigarette smoking, which can cause inflammation of the airways and also increase the mucus production in the nasal passages.*

▶ *Moderate your intake of alcohol, as it overrelaxes the muscles and tissues.*

▶ *Make sure that you get a good night's sleep every night. Going to bed when overtired will relax the muscles too much, making them sag and interfere with proper breathing.*

▶ *Reduce the stress in your life by taking up a relaxation routine.*

▶ *Relax before bedtime by sitting quietly or taking a warm bath. If you are not relaxed when you go to bed, there is more chance that your tissues will sag and exacerbate your snoring.*

HELPING TO PREVENT SNORING

Staying asleep at night can be difficult if you suffer from apnea. Some sufferers, on the other hand, find that they sleep throughout the night but wake up tired anyway because snoring has prevented them from entering a deep sleep. The techniques given below can help to prevent snoring.

▶ *Keep your evening meals light and don't eat too much just before you go to bed. Heavy food can cause your tissues and muscles to lose tone and interfere with your airways.*

▶ *Raise your head and shoulders above the bed with a firm pillow, preferably holding your jaw away from your body. You can also try sleeping on an incline by tilting the whole bed with boards or bricks under the legs at the head of the bed. This will help keep the airways open and allow you to breathe normally.*

▶ *Clear your nose and throat as completely as possible before you go to bed. Special nasal sprays are available from most pharmacies.*

▶ *Sleep on your stomach or your side. Sleeping on your back tends to aggravate snoring problems because most of the blockages are caused by the front of the throat and nasal passages relaxing downward.*

▶ *Obtain a special sleeping mask that blows air into the nose during the night and can help keep the airways open. They are very effective, although impractical for many users.*

▶ *Try a dental device that keeps your jaw forward and your tongue away from your throat to prevent airway blockage. A doctor or orthodontist needs to advise you and fit such a device.*

▶ *Consider surgery to widen the air passages in the throat if your case is very serious.*

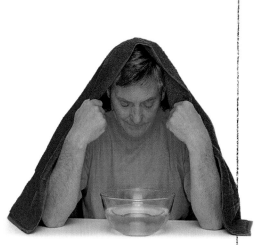

CLEARING YOUR PASSAGES
Make sure your nose and throat are clear of phlegm so they do not disrupt your breathing throughout the night. Nasal sprays and inhalants can both be used, as well as herbal inhalations.

SLEEPING WITH SOMEONE WITH A SNORING PROBLEM

If your partner has a severe snoring problem, you may find that your own sleep is suffering, perhaps more than your partner's, leaving you tired and agitated in the morning and putting a strain on your relationship. There are a number of steps you can take to ease the problem, although preventing the snoring altogether with one or other of the suggestions above would be the best solution because it would also help your partner sleep better.

▶ *Try gently pinching your partner's nose closed with your finger and thumb. It may encourage your partner to move into a better breathing position.*

▶ *If you can't stop the noise, try wearing earplugs so that you can't hear it.*

▶ *Concentrate on something else or perhaps even focus on the snoring itself; this tactic may help you forget what is preventing you from sleeping.*

▶ *Go to bed before your partner does so that you are in a deep sleep when he or she starts to snore.*

> **CAUTION**
> *Be careful when taking medications for snoring because they may prevent you from entering deep sleep, leaving you tired the following day. Likewise, if your partner's snoring is keeping you awake at night, sleeping pills are not a viable long-term solution.*

Raise the snorer's head to stop blockages in the throat.

Move the snorer onto his or her side or stomach to help prevent snoring.

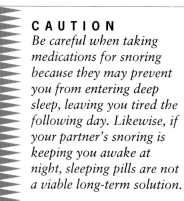

THE CORRECT POSITION
Make sure that your partner sleeps in the right position, on his or her side with the head slightly raised to open the air passages.

EMOTIONAL DRAIN ON ENERGY

Emotional stresses are among the most common causes of fatigue. Overwork, depression, an unhappy relationship, or anxiety can quickly deplete energy levels.

Low energy levels stemming from emotional problems tend to share certain features. Levels of activity diminish, and there is a reluctance to take on even simple tasks. Physical exertion, especially exercise, is often avoided, and an individual finds it increasingly difficult to participate even in pleasurable activities.

DEPRESSION

Depressive illness has been recognized for more than 2,000 years and, according to some experts, is the cause of more human misery than any other single disease. Depression accounts for an estimated 50 percent of psychiatric disorders and 5 to 10 percent of all visits to primary care doctors. Clinical depression is a severe manifestation of the problem and may require hospitalization in some cases.

Depression is often associated with a multitude of symptoms, including low spirits, irritability, lack of motivation, poor ability to concentrate, and sleep problems. However, it invariably includes fatigue and a general lack of vitality.

HOW DRUGS CAN AFFECT YOUR EMOTIONS

Neurons in the brain communicate with each other by means of neurotransmitters. These tiny chemicals are released from one neuron, pass through the synaptic gap, where their presence is experienced as a feeling, and are received by another neuron. Drugs have been developed to alter mood through the control of neurotransmitter efficiency. This is accomplished in one of three ways: by increasing the synthesis, or production, of neurotransmitters; by increasing the number of neurotransmitters released; or by releasing replica neurotransmitters that have a similar effect on the nervous system.

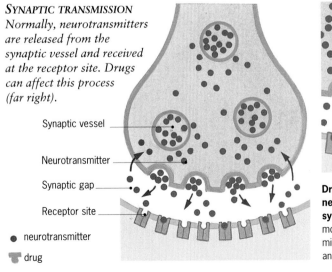

SYNAPTIC TRANSMISSION
Normally, neurotransmitters are released from the synaptic vessel and received at the receptor site. Drugs can affect this process (far right).

Synaptic vessel

Neurotransmitter

Synaptic gap

Receptor site

• neurotransmitter

drug

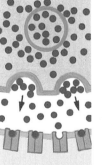

Drug increases neurotransmitter synthesis, so that more neurotransmitters are released and received.

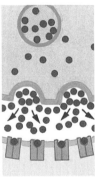

Drug increases release of neurotransmitters into the synaptic gap, and more are therefore received.

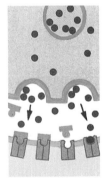

Drug contains artificial neurotransmitters, which activate receptor sites just as natural ones do.

A Perfectionist

Placing too many or too exacting demands on yourself can exhaust you both mentally and physically, reducing your energy levels and preventing you from functioning well. Clearing your head and taking time to relax can help you to get your life back into perspective, giving you the energy you need for a full and happy life.

Sebastian, 26, has always done well in school and expected a lot from himself. He has been working very hard to earn a doctorate in economics. Recently, however, he began feeling insecure about his work, especially after a progress meeting with his adviser, who suggested that parts of his thesis lacked depth. He has since been working long hours, researching and rewriting his thesis and drinking too much coffee to stay alert.

He is constantly tired but has difficulty sleeping. His girlfriend, Gail, has become increasingly concerned that he asks too much of himself. She thinks he has done enough to earn the doctorate, but Sebastian feels his work can still be improved and he cannot let it go.

WHAT SHOULD SEBASTIAN DO?

Gail suggested that Sebastian try cognitive behavioral therapy to help him put his perfectionist urges into perspective. This therapy looks for the underlying causes of ineffective or destructive attitudes and actions so that they can be addressed.

Such a therapist will ask Sebastian about his views on work, status, and achievement, as well as his upbringing, his own sense of self-worth, and performance anxieties. Together, they can work through Sebastian's inner anxieties and his expectations of both himself and those around him. The therapist will then make suggestions as to how he can alter his outlook, especially his negative reaction to criticism and his inability to relax.

Action Plan

STRESS
Take time off to relax, using meditation and yoga techniques. Spend more time in pleasurable activities to get more from life.

WORK
Don't overwork; take a break rather than working nonstop for hours at a time. Learn to be more realistic about expectations, goals, and deadlines.

EMOTIONS
Consider the reasons underlying behavior. Are they appropriate? Do they reflect Sebastian's own dreams or someone else's?

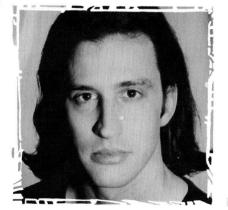

EMOTIONS
Many energy problems are caused by emotional difficulties that need to be resolved.

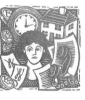

STRESS
Striving too hard for perfection or taking on too much can cause you to lose sight of your own personal goals and needs.

WORK
Working too hard and not allowing enough time to enjoy other aspects of life can lead to stress buildup.

HOW THINGS TURNED OUT FOR SEBASTIAN

The cognitive therapist quickly realized that Sebastian's perfectionism and hypercriticalness stemmed from his upbringing. The therapist helped him to see that he was unconsciously holding on to old behavioral patterns of seeking parental approval, which he no longer needed as an adult. He was encouraged to take up yoga, both to help himself relax and to increase his energy. He successfully completed his doctorate.

Finding your own path

Many parents have great ambitions for their children. Sometimes these reflect goals that they themselves could not achieve or a desire to maintain a family business or attain a certain status. Identifying and pursuing your own ambitions can be one of life's greatest challenges.

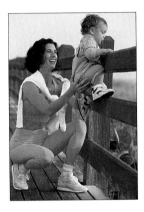

A GUIDING HAND
The best guidance that parents can give their children is to encourage them to stand on their own feet.

Depression often occurs as a reaction to a stressful situation that a person cannot cope with. This is called reactive depression. Grieving in response to the death of a spouse is one example. Another is the depression that follows a stroke or other serious physical illness. Depression is also common after childbirth, the so-called baby blues, or can result from hormonal disturbances, as in premenstrual syndrome. One of the best antidotes for reactive depression is to focus on daily routines to anchor yourself in reality. A funny movie or book may also improve your mood.

When depression occurs for no apparent reason, it is called endogenous. This form of depression, which tends to run in families, affects about 20 percent of women and 10 percent of men.

STRESS AND ANXIETY

A limited degree of stress and tension can be beneficial and actually boost energy levels and performance, helping to motivate individuals and spur them on to greater levels of achievement. But excessive stress and anxiety eat away at a person's vitality. They can create an energy vacuum, leading to poor health, greater anxiety, and a downward spiral of fatigue and low self-esteem that prevents the sufferer from leading a normal life.

One reason for this may be that prolonged stress can induce biological changes in a part of the brain called the hypothalamus,

ENERGY BOOST

Spring cleaning—even in the winter months—can be fun and revitalizing, brushing away the old cobwebs and making space for new pursuits and ideas. An interesting complementary therapy is space clearing, which is the spiritual cleansing of a room by clapping the hands together and ringing out the bad energy, neutralizing it for your own thoughts, ambitions, and enjoyment. Space clearing makes it possible to fill your personal space with positive feelings, building the foundations for an energized life.

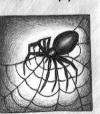

which, together with the pituitary gland, regulates hormone levels and autonomic functions, such as heart and breathing rate. The feelings of being hungry and of being satiated and the sensations of warmth and cold are located at specific centers in the hypothalamus; it is now believed that similar centers exist there for rest and fatigue. When the hypothalamus-pituitary system is disturbed by stress or depression, there is a consequent disruption in the normal regimen of activity and rest, resulting in fatigue, lethargy, and an inability to sleep.

OVERWORK AND BURNOUT

In today's society the pressure to succeed has become a major cause of stress and stress-related disorders and can ultimately lead to chronic fatigue and an inability to function well. Greater competition and increased media coverage of high achievers and status figures serve as inducements to push some people to their limits. Stress can manifest itself as a physical condition, such as a digestive problem, or as a nervous disorder, such as a mental breakdown.

Mental relaxation training is an important step in overcoming or avoiding the buildup of chronic stress. Relaxation techniques encourage a positive response to excess stress by decreasing heart rate and slowing breathing. Yoga is a form of exercise practiced for mental relaxation, and it may help relieve such disorders as insomnia, which can often be stress related.

Doing exercise and concentrating on your physical abilities can be surprisingly good for stress relief. Take your frustration out in a challenging squash competition or a strenuous aerobics class. Try a new dance class or play a game of soccer in the park with friends. Making fitness fun and inspiring can lift your spirits and help you overcome emotional problems, as well as stress.

Burnout

Burnout is a state of exhaustion in which a person feels physically and emotionally unable to do anything and may be suffering aches and illnesses as well. It usually results from prolonged stress and frustration and can be countered with relaxation.

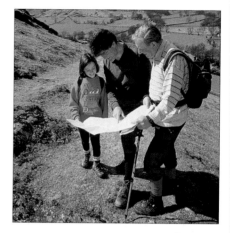

GET AWAY FROM IT ALL
Taking time off and getting away from your day-to-day life can help you put problems and pressures into perspective.

Many people suffer from burnout at some point in their lives, although they may not realize it themselves. Burnout occurs when your body is telling you that you need change. You have been working too hard at one part of your life, perhaps your job or caring for someone who is gravely ill and neglecting all else.

Every human being needs a balance of the emotional, social, intellectual, and practical aspects of life: denial or neglect of one leads to an imbalance that resounds throughout the whole. Many people who suffer from burnout are perfectionists in their work and feel that they are not getting enough support and appreciation from others, often because of isolation.

The warning signs of burnout include unexplained tiredness, irritability, difficulties in socializing and relaxing, and feelings of disenchantment, disorientation, cynicism, or sadness.

HELPING TO COPE WITH BURNOUT

There are a number of things you can do to reduce the risk of burnout or that will help you to cope if it should strike you down.

► *Admit that you have a problem. Make a conscious effort to change and focus on a number of measures to help yourself.*

► *Bring more variety into your life. Take up a new hobby or make time to relax with friends.*

► *Go away for a few days, even if your destination is not far from home. Get some fresh air and exercise. It is important to have a part of your life that is not goal oriented.*

► *If you know that you are a perfectionist, understand that people do make mistakes and need time and energy for a variety of things in life. Don't be a slave to your work or your goals.*

► *Accept your personal and emotional needs and limitations. If you don't have enough support or feedback, admit it to yourself and find the support you need.*

► *Regularly exercise and practice relaxation techniques (see Chapter 5) and take small breaks frequently to remind yourself what life is about in a wider context.*

TALK TO YOUR FAMILY AND FRIENDS
Many problems related to burnout can be positively addressed by opening up to someone close and giving that person the opportunity to share his or her own worries. Self-expression is one of the keys to good emotional health.

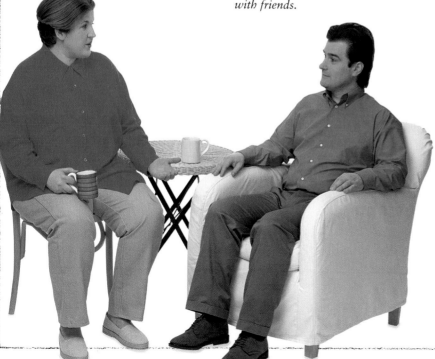

ALLERGIES AND INTOLERANCES

Occurring at any time of life, allergies and intolerances often cause fatigue and a loss of vitality. The situation may be compounded by difficulties in correctly diagnosing the cause.

Allergies and intolerances are common medical problems that can cause a wide range of symptoms, including fatigue. An allergy is an abnormal reaction by the immune system to substances that are perfectly harmless to other people. The immune system's function is to recognize a harmful foreign substance, such as a toxin or virus, and form antibodies to destroy it. Allergic reactions occur when the immune system mistakes harmless matter for an invader and builds up an army of antibodies to destroy it. This hypersensitivity can be a highly exaggerated and sometimes very dangerous response. An intolerance is also an abnormal reaction to a harmless substance, but it does not involve the immune system.

Some reactions are easy to diagnose because they occur in very specific situations or at particular times of the year. One example is hayfever, which a sufferer may notice is triggered by grass pollen and

DID YOU KNOW?

About half of all people who suffer a food intolerance have a craving for the very food that makes them unwell. It is thought that the offending food may have the side effect of increasing production of endorphins—the brain's natural painkillers that stimulate a good feeling. Intolerances to dairy or wheat products often cause this craving.

AVOIDING HIGH POLLEN COUNTS

For people who are allergic to pollen, understanding how and when different types of pollen are dispersed can help them to control the allergy. Tree pollen counts soar in April and May, grasses through June and July, and weed pollen is rife during August and September. Pollen levels also vary throughout the day.

POLLEN LEVELS THROUGHOUT THE DAY
Pollen is released in the morning and carried high in the air until late afternoon, when it falls back to the ground, sometimes many miles away. Sufferers of hayfever are advised against outdoor pursuits in the late afternoon, when pollen is returning to the ground.

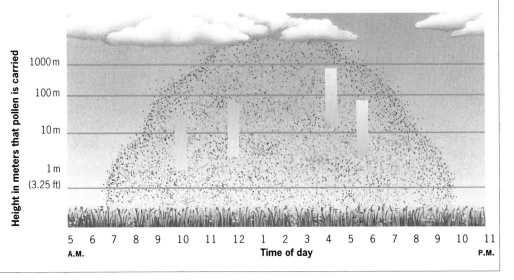

Height in meters that pollen is carried

1000 m
100 m
10 m
1 m
(3.25 ft)

5 6 7 8 9 10 11 12 1 2 3 4 5 6 7 8 9 10 11
A.M.   Time of day   P.M.

ALLERGIC TENSION-FATIGUE SYNDROME

This theory, developed in the United States in the 1930s, proposes that repeated exposure to an allergen exhausts the body, including the immune system, and leaves it open to illness and further medical complications. This can have a degenerative effect on energy levels, leading to chronic fatigue and serious health problems. Removing the allergen will improve not only the symptoms of the allergy but also the medical conditions caused by the drain on energy levels.

ALLERGIC DISORDERS AND FATIGUE

Although there are often a number of potential causes for any illness or condition, many symptoms can point to an undetected allergy. Allergies are one of the commonest causes of fatigue problems, but awareness of them may remain hidden for years. The culprits can usually be identified by using an allergy diary and having an allergy specialist test for reactions.

SYMPTOM	POSSIBLE CAUSE
Skin inflammation, eczema, dermatitis	House dust mites, laundry detergent, soap, body cream, cosmetics, fabric, stress, food
Respiratory problems, wheezing, asthma	Pollen, house dust mites, airborne pollution or dust particles, pet dander, mold spores, chemical fumes, food or beverage
Gastrointestinal disorders, vomiting, diarrhea, colic	Food or beverage, materials from cooking utensils, stress
Genitourinary disorders, candidiasis, cystitis	Tight or synthetic underclothing, laundry detergent, soap, douche, food or beverage

occurs only in the summer. In many cases, particularly where food is concerned, the cause of an allergy or intolerance can be difficult to establish.

SYMPTOMS OF ALLERGIES

Allergies and intolerances can cause a mixed and often confusing range of symptoms, including nausea, vomiting, migraine or other headaches, skin rash, ulcers, sinusitis, asthma, and muscle, bone, and joint pain. Behavioral problems are common, especially in children. They may include temper tantrums, screaming attacks, sulkiness, and ultrasensitivity. Adults may display fatigue, mood swings, anxiety, loss of sexual libido, and compulsive behavior.

The most serious form of allergic reaction is called anaphylactic shock. This is a potentially life-threatening condition involving severe facial redness and swelling, widespread itching and hives, difficulty breathing, a sudden drop in blood pressure, even unconsciousness. People at risk of anaphylactic shock should carry an emergency syringe of adrenaline, which, if administered promptly, can counteract shock.

ALLERGIES AND ENERGY LEVELS

Research carried out in Iceland in the early 1990s found that fatigue could be directly linked to allergy. In the study 200 people were tested for a specific and relatively common allergy to a wheat protein and were also tested for iron deficiency and a variety of symptoms, including fatigue. The 16 percent found to have the allergy also had slight deficiencies in iron, although none

were diagnosed as anemic, and they had complained of fatigue, headaches, and unexplained bouts of diarrhea to a significantly greater extent than those without the allergy. Researchers concluded that an allergy might cause many side effects, including fatigue, which could decrease quality of life without sufferers even knowing it.

A food allergy can be identified with one of three skin tests. Prick testing involves a tiny amount of the possible allergen being introduced into the superficial layer of skin. In intracutaneous testing, a larger dose of the allergen is injected directly into the dermis. This is a more sensitive test, although more uncomfortable and less practical than the prick test, and is primarily used as a follow-up. With a patch test, a plaster is doused with the allergen and affixed to the skin, which is then monitored for an allergic response.

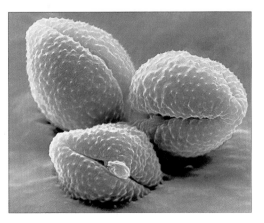

POLLEN
Under the microscope, pollen can be seen to have an aerodynamic shape that helps it to stay airborne. Pollen causes respiratory irritations when it enters the lungs of hayfever sufferers.

ENVIRONMENTAL FACTORS

The environments in which you live, work, and spend your free time can have an impact on your health. Revitalizing and healthful surroundings can greatly boost your energy.

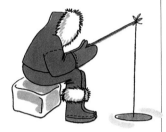

THE TOLLS OF TEMPERATURE
Extreme temperatures lower your energy and ability to work because your body is using much of its energy to adapt to the environment.

A number of different environmental factors can drain your energy without you even being aware of it. The most common problems are associated with buildings. Creating an indoor atmosphere conducive to energy and good health requires an understanding of the fundamental needs of people. A good supply of fresh air is of great importance for keeping oxygen levels high. Air free from pollutants is also important. Airborne pollutants such as dust, smoke particles, or gas fumes can all drain energy and, in the long run, cause major health risks, especially to the respiratory system.

Opening windows regularly, if possible, helps to keep air moving and reduces contamination from polluting paints, varnishes, and smoke, which contribute to environmental draining of energy. However, more subtle techniques, such as paying attention to furniture arrangment and decoration, can also boost energy. In the oriental art of Feng Shui, the furnishings in a room are used to enhance and direct energy in a positive way. The techniques are based on traditional Chinese theories of universal energy, or chi, and a system equating the directions of the compass with the different aspects of a person's nature and lifestyle.

Temperature factors
Temperature is another important element because activity levels are directly affected by heat and cold. The body's natural processes work best within a narrow band of temperatures. The best temperature for maximum energy is between 20° and 24°C (68° and 75°F). A temperature that is any cooler will cause you to use energy to keep warm; one that is warmer will make work more strenuous and draining.

Hot, humid weather is particularly debilitating because the body's main system of cooling itself—sweating—requires moisture to evaporate from the surface of the skin, but the high water content of the air makes this process more difficult, which can lead to rapid overheating. Of course, the effect of external temperatures can be compounded

---

COSMIC ENERGY FORCES: *The Wind*

In Scandinavian folklore the winds were said to be caused by a giant eagle that sat on the edge of heaven flapping its wings. In Scandinavia and other countries the wind was used by seafarers for thousands of years to power ships for transporting goods and people. Wind-powered transport reached its apotheosis in the sophisticated, multiple-sail tea clippers of the 19th century. Today wind is being used mainly for recreational sailing, but it is also being put to use on wind farms, where its power is harnessed by wind turbines and converted into electricity.

COMPUTER AND TV SCREENS

Looking at a computer or television screen for long periods can be highly stressful and cause headaches and muscular pains; it is especially tiring for the eyes. Office workers and others who spend long periods in front of a screen are advised to take frequent breaks to rest their eyes and to exercise the eyes regularly by looking across the room or out the window and focusing on a distant object. Similar techniques can help reduce eyestrain caused by excessive television viewing. Restricting viewing hours by getting out of the house and doing something active is often best.

by other factors. When doing strenuous physical work, for example, your body produces excess heat, which adds to the problem of overheating. Genetic makeup and physical characteristics such as skin color also help determine how quickly your body adjusts to climate changes.

Noise factors

Excessive or irritating noise can be very distracting and stressful and quickly become both physically and emotionally draining. Keeping irritating noise levels down can help to reduce energy-depleting stress. Playing soothing music or restful sounds like ocean waves or countryside noises softly in the background can have a positive effect on energy levels.

LIGHT

Light is a crucial element of life that has an important energizing effect on all living things. Getting the lighting right inside buildings can be difficult. Natural daylight is always preferable, but electric lighting is often needed to boost light levels during the day, as well as for nighttime illumination.

Constant low light levels can affect mood. A widely recognized condition is seasonal affective disorder (SAD), which is characterized by low energy and depression caused by lack of sunlight in the winter months. The condition particularly affects people in northern regions such as Scandinavia, where winter days are very short, but it is also known in places with less extreme winters. It

is not clearly understood why lack of sunlight has this effect, but the problem can be alleviated with daily exposure to specially formulated lights or by taking regular mini-vacations to a sunnier place.

There are many ways to enhance natural light and boost the energizing effect of your home. For example, you can place curtain rods to extend beyond a window so that when the curtains are open, they do not cover any part of it. You can position mirrors to reflect light from windows or add skylights to bring in additional light. Selecting light hues for walls and ceilings will also help make the most of available light.

The selection and placement of artificial light is also important. Lamps and overhead lighting should not glare and should be well situated for reading and other activities.

IN THE WORKPLACE

Environmental factors can greatly influence work output, and many companies have found that stress-related problems can be reduced through improvements in the work environment. Altering the light, humidity, noise, or temperature level, for example, has been shown to influence physical and mental performance and keep employees happier and less disturbed by external factors. This may be because of the effect of such factors on the hypothalamus, which monitors environmental conditions and alters energy output accordingly.

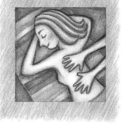

ENERGY BOOST

Treating yourself to a body massage can help soothe away tension. If you can't afford a professional masseur, enlist a friend, spouse, or family member.

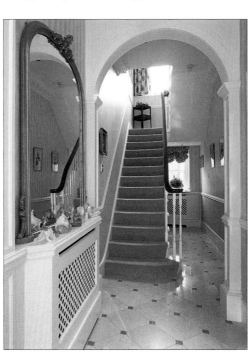

LETTING THE SUNLIGHT INTO YOUR LIFE
Making the most of natural light in your home through windows and skylights and the use of mirrors and pale colors in decoration can greatly enhance feelings of energy and warmth.

CHRONIC PAIN

Causing constant discomfort and distress, chronic pain drains energy as the body attempts to repair damage, compensate for impaired function, and cope with the pain itself.

Chronic pain is ongoing, lasting for months or even years, in contrast to acute pain, which is sudden and temporary. The long-term nature of chronic pain makes it particularly debilitating. One difficulty is the emotional and psychological strain imposed by trying to lead a normal and active life while handicapped by efforts to cope with constant suffering.

Lack of energy is often compounded by trying to compensate for the problem in the affected area and lessen the pain. Pain in the lower back, for instance, may prompt the sufferer to adopt an unnatural posture in order to take pressure off the problem area. Muscles that would normally be relaxed have to put in extra work and therefore use up more energy. This process also puts an excess load on neighboring muscles and joints that might be unused to it, thus causing further damage and pain in those areas. As a result, the sufferer feels exhausted merely from sitting, walking, or standing. People who suffer from osteoarthritis in the leg joints, for example, may find that a short walk is a major muscle-working exercise, demanding a rest afterward.

CHRONIC HEAD PAIN

Acute headaches usually result from tension in the head and neck muscles or inflamed blood vessels of the scalp and rarely last more than a few hours. They can be triggered by several factors, including noise, stress, hunger, and fatigue. Chronic head disorders cause prolonged stress, which is draining on energy reserves.

Migraines are a type of headache that can leave the sufferer bedridden for hours or even days. The throbbing pain is caused by spasms—the constriction and expansion—of blood vessels in the membranes (meninges) that surround the brain. They are often triggered by chemicals in such foods as citrus fruits, chocolate, cheese, and red wine, although stress, heightened emotional states, menstruation, and the contraceptive pill can also be causal factors.

PAIN IN THE JOINTS

Joint disorders such as osteoarthritis and rheumatoid arthritis can cause severe, chronic pain. Osteoarthritis is a condition in which the cartilage lining the joints breaks down, making movement difficult and painful. It usually affects the hips, knees, and spine and is most common in people aged 60

BOWEN TECHNIQUE

The Bowen technique is reputed to be highly beneficial for many types of physical pain. It incorporates a soft-tissue massage that works on the muscles, tendons, and ligaments very gently and with minimal pressure. The treatment can be performed with the patient wearing lightweight clothing, and no oils or special equipment are required. The gentleness of the therapy makes it ideal for treating elderly or very young people or when treatment would otherwise be difficult, perhaps because of a very recent and painful injury.

Regardless of the specific problem being treated, most people respond with a general energy boost, lessened pain, and a better outlook on life. The technique is wonderfully relaxing and can be useful in reducing stress.

The way the method works has been described by comparing the body to a light switch. The light and the switch may both be working, but if the wires are not connected properly, the light will not work. Bowen therapy helps to reestablish good connections between the body and brain.

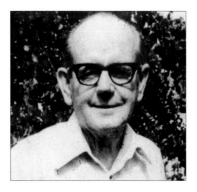

TOM BOWEN
Tom Bowen developed his special massage method in the 1950s and has since helped over 2,000 patients.

and older. Rheumatoid arthritis is an auto-immune disorder in which the immune system attacks the joints for no apparent reason. It can occur in any joint but most commonly affects the hands, wrists, feet, and ankles and may befall people of any age. In some cases food allergies or intolerances aggravate the symptoms.

Both forms of arthritis cause not only pain but usually swelling and stiffness as well. In advanced states, sufferers find any movement of the affected joints difficult and very painful, and the extra effort needed for movement drains energy.

BACK PAIN

Backache is one of the most common pain disorders. At least 80 percent of North Americans suffer an occasional backache, and for 15 percent the problem is chronic. Back problems are often the result of persistent bad posture; a sudden movement, like twisting, that strains the back muscles; or poor lifting technique, which can damage muscles or vertebrae. Stress is also thought to contribute to back problems because it causes muscular tension, which restricts flexibility and increases the risk of strains.

Such manipulative treatments as chiropractic, osteopathy, physiotherapy, and massage therapies have all proven effective in reliev-ing back pain. General relaxation techniques are also beneficial because they help relax the muscles and alleviate stress. People react differently to the various treatments available, however. Patients may need to try different approaches until they find the one that is most effective for them.

USING A PAIN DIARY

If you suffer from chronic pain, take a little time every day to make some notes about it. This will help you to build up a picture of what triggers your pain, what makes it better, and what makes it worse. First, describe how you feel on that particular day. Try to be as specific as possible; it does not matter if the words sound silly, just as long as you understand what you mean. Many people use a visual scale to compare how they feel from one day to the next. The scale goes from 0, meaning no pain, to 10, the worst pain experienced.

Make a note of what you ate each day and how it made you feel. This can help you to identify foods that make your condition worse. Write down as well any activities you undertook and how you felt afterward. This will allow you to draw on knowledge of previous situations before tackling something new. You may find that you are capable of more than you think.

Controlling pain
Researchers have found that pain can often be reduced by actively focusing attention on a nonpainful stimulus. For example, doing mental arithmetic exercises, such as counting backward by 25 from 1,000, or even singing a favorite song, can distract the brain from focusing on the pain.

PAIN PATHWAYS

When an excess of any type of stimulus is felt—for example, pressure, heat, or cold—the pain receptors under the skin signal the spinal cord by way of sensory neurons. The message is sent up the spinal cord to the thalamus, where impulses are sent into the parietal lobes. The individual now becomes aware of pain and can assess how best to respond.

PAIN TRANSMISSION
Different types of pain send different chemical messages to the brain, resulting in specific responses.

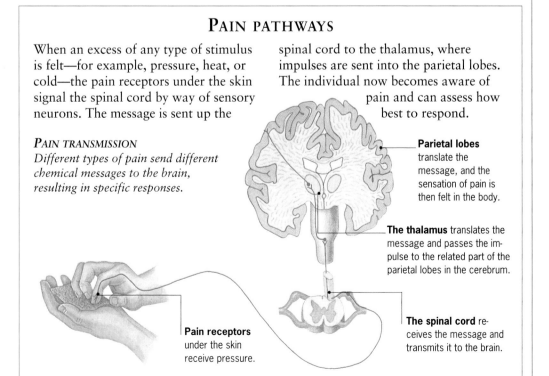

Parietal lobes translate the message, and the sensation of pain is then felt in the body.

The thalamus translates the message and passes the impulse to the related part of the parietal lobes in the cerebrum.

The spinal cord receives the message and transmits it to the brain.

Pain receptors under the skin receive pressure.

Natural Pain Beaters

Living with chronic pain presents a tough challenge to even the most positive of people. Natural pain relievers and careful adjustments in lifestyle can greatly increase energy levels and allow enjoyment of life despite the pain.

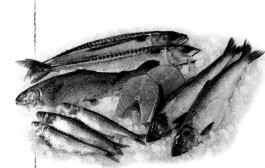

FISH OILS FOR ARTHRITIS
Fish oils contain omega-3 fatty acids, which are beneficial for arthritis. Good sources are (clockwise from top) herring, mackerel, sardines, trout, and salmon (center). Canned fish are not as beneficial because some of the oils are lost in the canning process.

Most people suffer occasional periods of pain, although these are usually temporary and easily forgotten. Others, however, live with ongoing or recurring pain, which can eat away at their energy and prevent them from enjoying a full life. Coping with this kind of pain is a two-step process. The first step is to come to terms with the pain and understand what is causing it. The second is to master the pain. This involves both physical treatments and mental control; it is necesary to think positively and not allow pain to rule.

Conventional medicine can offer complete or at least partial remission from pain for the short term, but all orthodox pain relievers have some unpleasant side effects; also, the body becomes less responsive to them over time. Natural remedies offer relief with fewer side effects, and most can be used indefinitely.

NATURAL THERAPIES

There are various natural therapies that can effectively ease pain and improve certain conditions; they can help to relax and soothe both body and spirit, allowing you to build up energy and restore well-being.

Touch therapies
There are a number of touch therapies, ranging from basic massage to more sophisticated physiotherapy techniques, that can be used to ease pain and aid recovery from injury. Some traditional touch therapies from Asia, which are becoming widespread in this country, can provide a more spiritual approach to pain relief. One of them is Tuina, a massage technique based on the power of the acupressure points. These are the gateways of the energy channels that pass through the body; when the points are pressed, energy flow may be improved,

SELF-MASSAGE
You can soothe your body at home with a relaxing self-massage. You don't need to massage your whole body but can focus on the part in which you feel discomfort. Certain acupressure points, held for a few minutes, are especially helpful for relieving pain.

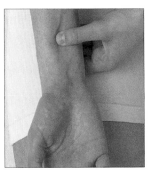 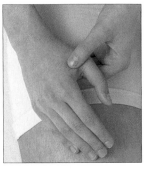

Pericardium 6 (P6) is a powerful point that is used for nausea, emotional pain, and anxiety and is also good for strengthening the heartbeat. The point is located three finger widths above the wrist between the two large tendons.

Large Intestine 4 (L4) is good for inducing calmness and well-being. It keeps elimination regular and stimulates the immune system as well. (This point must not be used during pregnancy because it may stimulate premature contractions.) It is located at the base of the V formed between the thumb and index finger.

promoting better health, vitality, and balance. Other Eastern touch therapies that work on energy levels in a similar way are shiatsu and Jin Shin, both of which originated in Japan.

Yet another system, Reiki, involves passing healing energy from a healer to a patient; the healer places his or her hands on the patient's body and concentrates on the transfer.

Thai massage is a vigorous system, with the therapist bending and manipulating the patient through a number of movements and positions.

Three other manipulative therapies are osteopathy, chiropractic, and physiotherapy. They are well established within the medical framework and are often connected to hospitals or doctors' clinics. Osteopathy and chiropractic both aim to restore the proper alignment of the body, particularly the spine, in order to rebalance the body and restore it to

health. Physiotherapy involves a number of techniques, including ultrasound and hydrotherapy, to promote tissue repair and proper functioning of the body.

Dietary considerations

A diet that includes a wide variety of foods, a large proportion of which are fruits and vegetables, can help alleviate a number of health problems and prevent the onset or worsening of many more. The key is to keep it balanced; an excess of any one nutrient can cause a negative value of another. (See Chapter 4 for the daily requirements of nutrients that are especially important for maintaining high energy levels.)

Avoid refined sugar, which can disrupt the balance of energy, and cut down on fats because they tend to aggravate health problems. Saturated fats, in particular, can lead

to cardiovascular disorders. Also, try to keep your weight within normal limits. Being either overweight or underweight will aggravate many medical conditions, and obesity can lead to severe energy problems that will hinder recovery.

Positive thinking

Try to perceive your body as a whole entity that encompasses both the pain and the parts that function well and try to put the pain into context. Remember that you are an energized being with the power to achieve what you want. Becoming a slave to pain is all too easy; shun it by taking control of your life and not letting pain get you down. Also, work on ways to obtain a good night's sleep without the use of sleeping pills or drugs (see pages 54–59). Sleep will always help you recover your energy and leave you feeling refreshed.

NATURAL PAINKILLERS

Herbal remedies have been used for thousands of years to combat pain and ease disorders. Some of the more time-tested remedies are listed below, but you should check with your doctor before trying them if you have a serious condition.

PROBLEM	HERBAL REMEDY	PREPARATION
Stomach ulcers	Licorice	Drink herbal infusion.
Indigestion	Meadowsweet, Marsh mallow, Peppermint, Fennel, Cinnamon	Drink herbal infusion or eat as sweets.
Nausea	Ginger, Horehound	Drink herbal infusion.
Constipation	Yellow dock	Drink herbal infusion.
Diarrhea	Agrimony	Drink herbal infusion.
Breathing problems	Thyme, Eucalyptus	Inhale a hot infusion.
Menstrual pain	Chamomile, Peppermint	Drink herbal infusion.
Throat problems	Agrimony, Sage	Use infusion as a gargle.
Headache	Vervain	Place cold compress with an infusion on back of neck.
Muscle damage	Wintergreen	Apply to skin, mixed with 4 parts oil.
Rheumatic pain	Red pepper, Eucalyptus, Clove	Apply to skin.
Muscle pain	St. John's wort, Lavender	Apply to skin.
Arthritis	Chamomile, Juniper, Wintergreen	Apply to skin.

Thyme, prepared as a tea, is good for breathing problems.

Rosemary can be used in creams and massage oils for arthritis.

Sage tea can be used as a gargle to ease sore throat.

Clove oil may help relieve rheumatic pain.

DIETS THAT DRAIN ENERGY

If you are not getting the correct balance of fuel and nutrients from your food, you may find yourself feeling lethargic and lacking vitality.

HEALTHY EATING

Adopting the following dietary tips can help improve your health.

► *Cut the fat off meat.*

► *Buy low-fat versions of dairy products.*

► *Broil, steam, poach, or roast food instead of frying it.*

► *Avoid highly refined or processed foods.*

► *Eat at least two pieces of fresh fruit every day.*

► *Have a varied diet.*

► *Avoid sugary foods.*

► *Cook vegetables with as little water and for as little time as possible.*

EMPTY CALORIES
Fruits and vegetables have more nutrients per calorie than most fast foods made with high fat and refined ingredients.

Food is the fuel that drives the engine of the human body. The role that many of food's nutrients, including vitamins and minerals, play in keeping us healthy and preventing disease has been well documented. Although there is still much to learn and some controversy remains over the amounts of certain nutrients that humans need for optimum health, sufficient knowledge exists to provide basic guidelines you can follow to ensure that your diet is providing all the energy you need.

NUTRITIONAL DEFICIENCY
The absorbing of food depends on a complex pattern of chemical reactions and interactions. Since proper functioning of the body requires a combination of many nutrients, a deficiency of even one can result in loss of energy, as well as other problems.

A varied and well-balanced diet will usually provide the body with everything it needs in the right proportions. There are situations, however, that call for an increase in nutrients to maintain optimum health and energy levels. For example, any disorder that causes repeated vomiting or diarrhea can quickly deplete the body of vital trace elements and also prevent it from

extracting all the nourishment available in food. It may be necessary to increase the intake of some vitamins and minerals to compensate. People who have suffered a severe injury or burn or undergone surgery also need extra nutrients to help their body tissues repair themselves

The elderly are at particular risk for nutritional deficiencies because their ability to absorb certain nutrients is diminished and their appetites are often poor as well.

Many women suffer from iron deficiency anemia because large amounts of this mineral, a major component of red blood cells, is lost during menstruation. Anemia is typically characterized by reduced energy levels. In addition to extra iron, women who are pregnant or nursing need more than the average daily requirements of other nutrients to support the growth of the child without depleting their own nutritional stores. More information about energy-linked nutrients can be found in Chapter 4.

DIETING AND WEIGHT CONTROL
Fatigue is a common problem for people who are trying to lose weight, particularly if they are not following a well-balanced diet. Problems arise mainly when a dieter wants

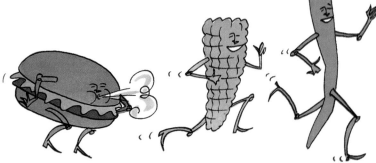

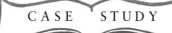

A Caffeine Addict

Using caffeine to wake up in the morning and keep going during the day can lead to an ever-growing need for more caffeine and, eventually, nagging fatigue and a headache when caffeine is unavailable. It can also result in jitteriness and irritability. Reducing caffeine gradually and maintaining a healthy diet and regular sleeping pattern can help rebalance natural energy levels.

Damien is a newspaper reporter in his late twenties. He has recently been promoted and has found it difficult to keep up with his new workload. This is compounded by an active social life that involves drinking with friends many evenings. In order to get through his work, he has been going to the office earlier in the morning and drinking large doses of strong coffee to boost his alertness. He has felt himself becoming increasingly exhausted, however, and is depending more and more on caffeine to stay awake during the day.

He can see that a vicious circle of insufficient sleep and coffee addiction is starting to affect his whole life adversely. A concerned colleague has advised him to do something before he has a nervous collapse.

WHAT SHOULD DAMIEN DO?

Damien needs to regain control over his habits and alter his lifestyle. Although initially skeptical, he went to see a practitioner of traditional Chinese medicine. The doctor explained how Damien's excessive use of caffeine was actually making his exhaustion worse in the long run. He recommended that Damien revise his drinking and social habits and forgo coffee. Cutting back on caffeine may be difficult at first but, in the long run, it will allow Damien's natural energy levels to improve. The practitioner recommended a program of acupuncture and herbal treatments to help Damien overcome his caffeine addiction and counter the stress factors in his life.

HEALTH
Too little sleep and too much alcohol make large demands on energy levels.

DIET
Drinking too much coffee can boost energy temporarily but leads to fatigue in the long term.

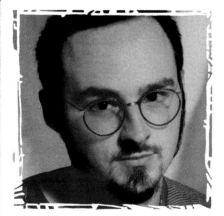

LIFESTYLE
Keeping up a hectic social life can leave you lacking vitality for work.

Action Plan

HEALTH
Cut down on alcohol consumption to improve sleep. Get into the habit of going to bed and getting up at regular times and strive for eight hours of sleep each night.

DIET
Resist the urge to get a quick energy boost with caffeine; it will sap Damien's energy in the long run and leave him needing more.

LIFESTYLE
Restrict drinking with friends to the weekends and keep weekdays free for work, relaxation, and good sleep. Give up smoking.

HOW THINGS TURNED OUT FOR DAMIEN

At first Damien missed both his coffee and his regular nights out, although the acupuncture gradually helped him relax and overcome his coffee cravings. After a few weeks he felt his energy levels starting to improve. Soon he was mentally and physically alert throughout the day at work. He has joined a gym, and his twice-weekly workouts have boosted his energy levels even more. He really looks forward to his social events on the weekends.

to lose weight quickly, perhaps for a wedding, and cuts down food intake severely in a "crash" diet. Generally, a crash diet does not provide enough readily available energy to meet the body's basic requirements, and it often lacks vital vitamins and minerals. In such diets the available energy stores are used quickly, leaving only the long-term fat stores to fuel the body. Because these are not so readily converted into energy, the dieter may feel lethargic and experience headaches, digestive upsets, and depression. The body's basal metabolic rate also slows down as an emergency measure to protect the body against starvation. This slows the rate at which stored fat is used and makes the diet less effective for losing weight.

The body needs a certain level of energy in order to burn up fat stores. A nutritionist or dietitian will take this into account when planning a diet for you, as well as ensuring that your meals have adequate levels of vitamins and minerals. A properly planned weight-loss diet is both healthier and more efficient than a crash diet.

Long-term restrictive diets can also be detrimental to energy levels unless they are carefully monitored. Vegetarians, especially vegans (who eat no animal products at all), can enjoy perfect health but need to take special care to obtain sufficient protein, iron, and vitamin B_{12}.

People who have difficulty absorbing or tolerating certain foods, such as wheat or milk, are also at risk for being malnourished because they have to exclude these foods from their diet. These exclusions can lead to greatly reduced energy levels and possible

EXTRA-HEALTHY DIET
The "Mediterranean diet" is considered to be one of the world's healthiest. It is based largely on pasta, rice, bread, and other grain foods, accompanied by ample vegetables and fruits and modest amounts of meat and seafood. Legumes, nuts, seeds, and olive oil are also used in abundance, and wine often accompanies lunch and dinner.

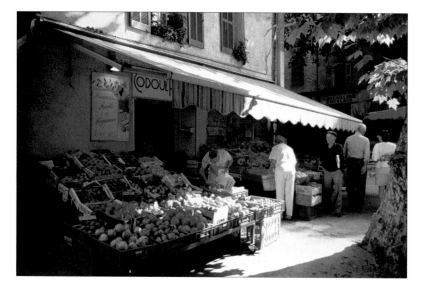

Origins

The condition of anemia was first identified by a German physician, Dr. Johannes Lange, who wrote a paper in 1554 entitled "Concerning the Disease of the Virgins." He described the weakness and fatigue suffered by young women as characterized by shortness of breath and poor appetite. Lange named the condition "chlorosis" because the sufferer's complexion was usually pale and tinged with green.

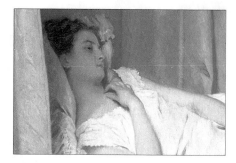

CHLOROSIS
This anemic condition was once romantically associated with young women, depicted as weak and prone to fainting.

health disorders in the long term unless a diet is planned carefully to compensate for the foods that must be avoided.

OVERWEIGHT

Most calories that are not converted right away into energy for powering bodily processes or physical activities are stored as fat. An overaccumulation of fat can affect energy levels in several ways. The strain of carrying excess weight makes people become breathless and tire faster, and they tend to become less mobile as a result. This lack of movement reduces the amount of energy burned, so even more calories are stored as fat. Excess fat can lead to serious health problems, such as raised blood pressure and heart disease. The downward spiral continues until the excess weight is lost.

Being overweight is a big health problem in the United States, affecting just over half of all adults. Of these, 30 percent are obese, defined as being more than 20 percent above the ideal weight for height, build, and age. In Canada 30 percent of adults between 20 and 64 are overweight; about 4 percent of the population is obese, which Canadians define as a Body Mass Index (BMI) of 30 or greater. (The BMI is calculated by dividing a person's weight in kilograms by his or her height in meters squared.)

Some experts believe that not only the additional weight but also its distribution is linked to health problems. For example, excess abdominal fat carries a greater risk than fat in the hips and thighs because the liver converts more abdominal fat into types that circulate in the bloodstream and can form the plaque in clogged arteries.

In addition to physical problems, being overweight often carries a social stigma. This can deter fat people from leaving their homes and lead to an even greater lack of mobility and a buildup of unused fat stores, as well as lack of self-esteem and increased social isolation.

Appetite and behavior

A number of studies have established links between being overweight, overeating, and feeling satisfied with the amount of food eaten. Overweight has been revealed as a very complex issue, involving metabolism, genetic makeup, and emotional and psychological factors, as well as the type and amount of food consumed. Some research with animals suggests that when food is both rich in protein and highly palatable, more than the necessary amount will be eaten.

A strong relationship has also been found between emotions and appetite. For example, appetite tends to increase during times of stress, anxiety, and low mood, whereas maintaining a relaxed, calm state of mind tends to stabilize or decrease appetite.

Obesity has been called a disease of food abuse and can sometimes be tackled by checking the impulse for binge eating. There are practical tips you can follow to avoid excess eating. They include drinking plenty of water before and during meals to help fill up the stomach, putting meals on smaller plates so you are not tempted to serve yourself too much, chewing more slowly and pausing longer between mouthfuls to allow food time to go down, avoiding sugary and high-fat snacks between meals, filling up with fruits and vegetables, and getting up from the table before you are full. It can also help to consume most of your calories during the day and have a light meal in the evening.

It is important to realize that people often eat not just because they are hungry but because of social situations. For instance, a considerable amount of overeating is related to dining out—whether for business reasons or with friends—when multiple courses may be eaten out of custom rather than hunger. Business lunches are a particular problem because the host may feel compelled to show generosity by encouraging guests to select several courses.

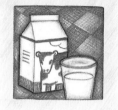

YIN AND YANG FOODS

Traditional Chinese medicine promotes a balance between yin, the female force, and yang, the male force. Diet plays a major role in balancing these energies by subduing overactive energies with foods from the opposite energy.

Yang foods include meat, fish, cooked vegetables, nuts, and beans

Yin foods include watermelon and other soft fruits, bamboo shoots, honey, chili peppers, and lemons.

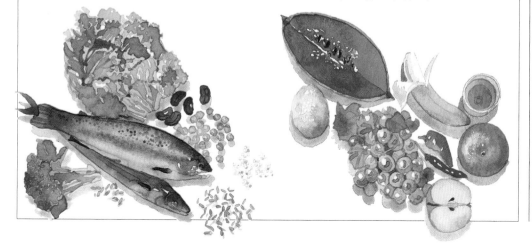

Daytime Drowsiness

Drowsiness during the day can be disruptive to work and even dangerous for people who are driving vehicles or operating heavy machinery. There are a number of ways to avoid or curb daytime drowsiness.

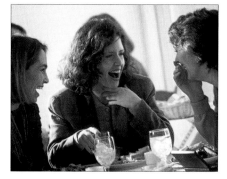

HAVE SOME FUN
Balancing work with fun can help you to stay alert and active. Also, taking on a variety of assignments rather than plodding away at just one lengthy task can keep your motivation up.

Feelings of drowsiness can affect people in different ways; some feel drained or find it difficult to concentrate, whereas others drop into a light sleep after a meal. However it affects you, daytime drowsiness can disrupt your ability to get on with a normal life.

Many factors can cause daytime drowsiness, including poor sleep at night, an inadequate diet, or a more serious condition or illness. It is important initially to try to locate the cause of the drowsiness. In this chapter and Chapter 6, some of the common problems and conditions associated with fatigue are described and explained. If you think that you may be suffering from a more serious illness, you should see your doctor. You should also seek the advice of a doctor if your drowsiness continues after you have tried the suggestions below and opposite.

ORGANIZING YOUR LIFE TO PREVENT DROWSINESS

One way to maintain a steady flow of energy is to listen to your body's needs and avoid or offset periods of sagging energy by planning your life to accommodate them. If, for instance, your body slows down at certain times of the day, allow time to rest or do low-key activities for that particular period, or have a nourishing snack to restore flagging energy. If a heavy lunch makes you sleepy, eat lightly at midday. If insomnia is robbing you of sleep, see page 55 for ways to deal with it.

STRETCHING
If you find yourself getting sleepy, taking a good stretch will usually get your blood flowing. This exercise helps the blood flow to your head, revitalizing your mind.

Keep your back as straight as you can.

Straighten your legs and keep your feet shoulder width apart for support.

ENERGIZING TIPS

Taking time to better organize your life can help you to find energy when you need it.

▶ *Consider your energy priorities. Make a list of all the things that you need to do and then list them in order of priority. If you do not have the energy to do everything, see if the items at the bottom can be delegated or eliminated or done less frequently.*

▶ *Do not waste energy on worrying. People often lose sleep and suffer from tiredness during an anxious period. Instead, focus on finding a solution and enlisting other people's help if necessary.*

▶ *Take a brisk walk to get some fresh air into your lungs and increase your heartbeat. This will speed the flow of blood around your body, enabling you to think, move, and react faster. Usually a 10-minute walk is all that is needed for revitalizing the body and mind.*

DRINKS AND YOUR ENERGY LEVELS

Many people ignore the health aspects of beverages, although they can play a major part in providing energy—good examples are milk shakes and juices—or in reducing it—sodas and alcoholic drinks are culprits. The adult body needs about 2 liters (2 quarts) of fluid every day to keep the body energized.

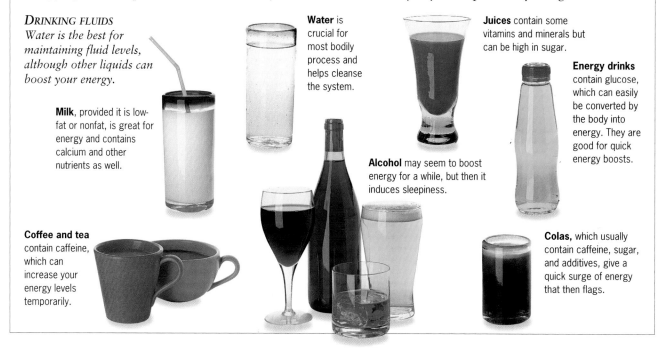

DRINKING FLUIDS
Water is the best for maintaining fluid levels, although other liquids can boost your energy.

Milk, provided it is low-fat or nonfat, is great for energy and contains calcium and other nutrients as well.

Coffee and tea contain caffeine, which can increase your energy levels temporarily.

Water is crucial for most bodily process and helps cleanse the system.

Alcohol may seem to boost energy for a while, but then it induces sleepiness.

Juices contain some vitamins and minerals but can be high in sugar.

Energy drinks contain glucose, which can easily be converted by the body into energy. They are good for quick energy boosts.

Colas, which usually contain caffeine, sugar, and additives, give a quick surge of energy that then flags.

DIETARY ADVICE

Keeping your diet healthy and well balanced will help you tackle daytime drowsiness. Make a note of times during the day when you feel tend to feel sleepy, then plan to counteract the tiredness with an energy-providing snack or beverage.

▶ *If possible, avoid eating heavy meals because your energy will be focused on digesting the food. This is often the reason that people fall asleep after a heavy lunch.*

▶ *Eat smaller, more frequent meals throughout the day. This regimen is better at keeping energy levels steady.*

▶ *Make complex carbohydrates (starches) and fruits and vegetables the main constituents of your diet. These provide a readily used source of energy plus the nutrients and fiber you need.*

▶ *Avoid sugary snacks and foods; they may give you a quick energy fix, but this surge will soon wear off, leaving you more tired than before.*

▶ *Drink a cup of tea or coffee. Researchers in Massachusetts found that the caffeine in one cup of coffee can*

provide an energy boost that lasts for up to six hours. However, you should limit your intake to two cups a day; more than this amount can cause insomnia and reduce the body's absorption of certain minerals. Also, keep in mind that coffee contains more caffeine than tea.

ENERGY SNACKS
You can boost your energy throughout the day by having nourishing snacks. However, you should avoid snacks that contain refined sugar and fat and focus on those high in complex carbohydrates, nutrients, and fiber.

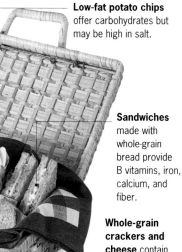

Low-fat potato chips offer carbohydrates but may be high in salt.

Bananas make good potassium-rich snacks.

Cereal bars contain B vitamins and fiber but may be high in fat.

Yogurt has vitamins B_2 and B_{12}, as well as friendly bacteria.

Nuts contain B and E vitamins and minerals.

Dried fruit is a good source of iron and potassium.

Sandwiches made with whole-grain bread provide B vitamins, iron, calcium, and fiber.

Whole-grain crackers and cheese contain protein, calcium, and vitamin B_{12}.

Apples provide some vitamins and minerals plus fiber.

DRUGS THAT DRAIN ENERGY

Medicinal drugs can affect energy levels in different ways, for example, by acting on brain cells or by altering hormone levels and chemical makeup.

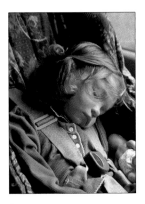

FATIGUE FACTOR
Travel sickness pills, often given to children, can cause drowsiness.

Medicines, both prescription and over-the-counter, are an integral part of the way we deal with illness and health maintenance. However, we have to keep in mind that chemical changes and emotional disturbances caused by drugs can sometimes lead to a chain reaction that affects energy levels. These effects can be compounded when one drug is combined with another medication or with food.

PRESCRIPTION DRUGS

There are a large number of prescription drugs that can make you feel tired and lethargic, often because of their influence on neurotransmitters in the brain. This effect may be even more marked when a drug is

taken in combination with over-the-counter preparations, other prescription drugs, alcohol, or foods such as milk. For this reason it is important to ask your doctor about possible side effects and find out whether certain substances may cause complications when you are taking the medication.

Some antidepressants trigger the release of chemicals in the brain that stimulate nerve activity that may lead to fatigue, lethargy, and drowsiness. Similarly, some antipsychotic medications, used to alleviate severe anxiety and other problematic mental states, can cause lethargy and drowsiness. This is because they work by blocking the action of dopamine, a natural chemical in the brain that stimulates nerve action.

Antiepileptic drugs, which inhibit electrical activity within the brain to prevent seizures, can reduce mental alertness. Some drugs that are used to lower blood pressure can also cause dizziness and fainting. Antivomiting drugs, which reduce nerve activity at the base of the brain to suppress the vomiting reflex, cause drowsiness as well.

Sleeping pills and tranquilizers are no longer prescribed as readily as they used to

PAIN-RELIEVING DRUGS

Many drugs that are used for relieving pain have possible side effects that can greatly influence your energy levels. Always read and follow the instructions for them carefully.

DRUG	POSSIBLE COMMON SIDE EFFECTS
Acetaminophen	No common side effects, but prolonged use may lead to liver problems, kidney problems, or anemia.
Aspirin	Stomach upset, rash, nausea, ringing in the ears
Codeine	Dizziness, nausea, constipation, drowsiness, addiction
Ibuprofen	Nausea, heartburn, diarrhea, dizziness, sleepiness
Diclofenac	Nausea, heartburn, dizziness, constipation, sleepiness
Naproxen	Nausea, vomiting, heartburn, diarrhea, constipation dizziness, sleepiness
Fentanyl	Dizziness, constipation, nausea, itching, addiction
Morphine	Drowsiness, dizziness, constipation, nausea, addiction

ANTIDEPRESSANTS

Used to improve mood, antidepressants such as Prozac increase the neurotransmitter serotonin in the brain, speeding the transport of information. This helps to lift people out of their depression, allowing them to take a more detached approach to problems and to resolve anxieties. At the same time it can cause inability to concentrate and tiredness, although the positive feelings usually counteract any bad effects. The drug takes four to six weeks to work, and the wait can sometimes worsen the depression. Likewise, coming off the drug can be difficult because the body may have stopped producing normal levels of serotonin naturally. This often leads to more depression and an inability to function properly.

be because it was realized that they interfere with the normal sleeping patterns necessary for good physical and mental health. They can also be highly addictive, leading to tolerance, dependency, and an inability to sleep properly without the drug.

Drugs and food interactions

Some common foods, especially cheese, wine, grapefruit, and tea, can interact with prescription drugs and either block or intensify their effects. Cheese and wine contain monoamines, which have a similar chemical structure to that of some amphetamines; when mixed with drugs, they may cause nightmares, migraines, hallucinations, and raised blood pressure. It is the monoamines in cheese that are thought to cause nightmares in some people.

Grapefruit reduces the effect of an enzyme in the small intestine that breaks down medications, increasing the amount that is absorbed by the body. Those taking drugs for hayfever and heart disorders are warned not to eat grapefruit, and some research suggests that women taking the contraceptive pill should also avoid eating the fruit, although this advice remains controversial.

Tea and coffee contain substances that can reduce the absorption of some vitamins and minerals, particularly iron. It is advisable to allow a gap of at least an hour following a meal or after taking supplements before drinking tea or coffee to ensure the proper absorption of nutrients.

OVER-THE-COUNTER DRUGS

Many over-the-counter drugs can alter your energy levels, making you tired, lethargic, and unable to concentrate, although some remedies include caffeine or other stimulants to counteract this effect. Cold and hayfever remedies, in particular, often contain antihistamines for relieving a runny nose. Because they can cause drowsiness and make it dangerous to operate machinery or drive an automobile, their use in the daytime should be avoided.

Acetaminophen, one of the most popular medications for controlling pain and lowering fever, has few side effects. It does not alter energy levels; however, the risk of accidental overdose is high. Combining different medications that include acetaminophen should be avoided.

Aspirin is another popular painkiller and antipyretic and, unlike acetaminophen, it can also relieve inflammation. But aspirin can cause stomach bleeding if taken for long periods and so is unsuitable for those suffering from gastrointestinal disorders. It is not recommended for anyone with asthma or children under 12, except on a doctor's advice.

THE CONTRACEPTIVE PILL

Although many women enjoy the positive benefits of the contraceptive pill, some find that it drains their energy. The contraceptive pill works by altering hormone levels in the body to mimic those of pregnancy, and many of the side effects are similar to the symptoms, including tiredness, that are experienced during the early part of pregnancy. If you think the pill may be causing energy problems, you may prefer to take the progesterone-only pill, which has fewer side effects, although it is slightly less reliable.

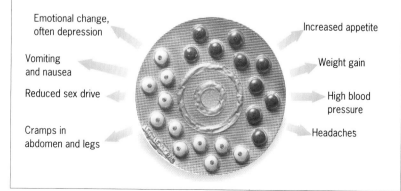

Emotional change, often depression

Vomiting and nausea

Reduced sex drive

Cramps in abdomen and legs

Increased appetite

Weight gain

High blood pressure

Headaches

DRUGS AND COMPETENCE

Many commonly used drugs can greatly affect your ability and motivation to work. The benefits from them are widely utilized, such as the energy boost from caffeine and the relaxing effect of alcohol. However, if you have a job to do, you should consider the side effects of any substances you intend to take.

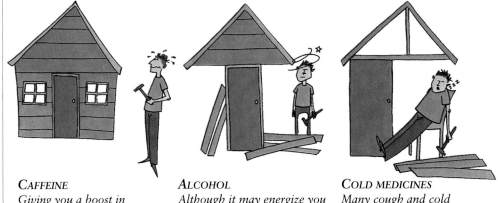

CAFFEINE
Giving you a boost in alertness and energy, caffeine can later leave you tired.

ALCOHOL
Although it may energize you briefly, alcohol can prevent you from performing well.

COLD MEDICINES
Many cough and cold remedies make you feel relaxed and lethargic.

Ibuprofen is a painkiller and anti-inflammatory with fewer side effects than aspirin. It is particularly useful for menstrual pains and rheumatoid arthritis. In susceptible individuals, however, it can cause lethargy, nausea, and other digestive disorders.

Codeine, a narcotic painkiller derived from the opium poppy, is often combined with other painkillers. It may make you drowsy, so don't plan anything strenuous.

NICOTINE

Nicotine is a stimulant found in tobacco that is usually taken in through the lungs by smoking the plant's leaves. The predominant effects are on the autonomic nervous system, which controls such automatic, involuntary body functions as heart rate and breathing. The drug works in different ways from person to person. Someone not used to nicotine will experience a lowering of the heart rate, whereas a nicotine addict will have an increased heartbeat and raised blood pressure. Nicotine also stimulates the central nervous system, increasing alertness and improving concentration, but it is addictive; users need progressively larger amounts to stimulate their system.

ALCOHOL

Alcohol depresses the central nervous system, decreasing the activity of the brain and reducing anxiety, tension, and inhibitions. It is used widely throughout most of the world for its relaxing effects, and in small quantities it may help to relieve stress temporarily. However, performance rapidly deteriorates with increased alcohol intake because it impairs both mental and physical functions. It has a slight stimulant effect that can delay the onset of fatigue for a while, but continued drinking causes sleepiness and sometimes even unconsciousness. The following day you may find yourself dehydrated and unable to concentrate.

STEROID DRUGS

Anabolic steroids are sometimes taken by bodybuilders and athletes to increase muscle size and thus energy potential. They are derived from the male hormone testosterone and can cause aggressive behavior and side effects that influence the characteristics and sexual functioning of a person.

RECREATIONAL DRUGS

Some people take "recreational" drugs to change their mood and energy levels. Some of these drugs are also used in a psychiatric framework to study the workings of the human mind and to help individuals to express their anxieties and deeper emotional worries. However, most are not conducive in the long term to good physical and psychological health, and they often entail withdrawal symptoms that reduce energy.

CHAPTER 4

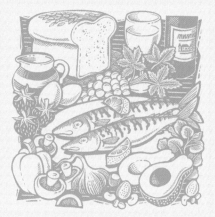

EATING FOR ENERGY

Numerous studies have clearly shown the important part that diet plays in preventing disease and illness. If you understand the essential components of healthy eating, as well as the role that particular nutrients have in energy production, you can eat to optimize your health and energy.

THE COMPONENTS OF HEALTHY EATING

Energy comes directly from the food that you eat, so if you understand the basic elements of healthy eating, improved well-being and vitality will be within your grasp.

Energy is needed by the human body to function normally. The energy is obtained from the major components of food—carbohydrates, protein, and fat—and is measured in calories by weight. Carbohydrates and protein provide 4 calories per gram; fat provides 9 calories per gram.

The body produces energy in much the same way as a train engine; fuel is used to feed a process that releases energy as a product. The essential difference between the two is that in the body, energy is released gradually in a series of steps, each carefully controlled by enzymes and hormones. This energy can then be used as needed for movement and vital processes.

CARBOHYDRATES

Of the three main nutrients, carbohydrates provide energy for immediate use; the body converts them to glucose, or blood sugar. At any given time the blood can carry enough glucose to last about an hour. Any carbohy-

YOUR DAILY DIET

For the best of health and vitality, a balanced diet that consists mainly of complex carbohydrates, fruits, and vegetables is advised. Cutting fats and sugars down to a small portion of your daily food intake and keeping animal foods to a minimum will also be of benefit.

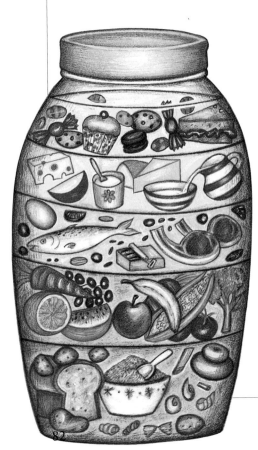

BASIC DIET
A balanced diet consists of a variety of foods consumed in optimum quantities.

Foods containing fat and sugar should be kept to a minimum. Snacks often contain surprisingly large amounts of unhealthy saturated fats.

Milk and dairy foods should be eaten in moderation. Choose lower-fat alternatives.

Meat, fish, and poultry should be eaten in moderate amounts. If you are vegetarian, include more beans, nuts, and seeds in your diet.

Fruit and vegetables should provide a good proportion of your diet. The minimum goal is five portions a day, not including potatoes.

Bread, other grain foods, and potatoes should provide the bulk of your diet. If you are dieting, cut down on fat and sugar, not grains.

THREE DIET RULES

The World Health Organization (WHO) recommends following the three rules below to help reduce the incidence of heart disease and cancer.

▶ *For at least half of your food, choose starchy carbohydrates such as bread, pasta, rice, and potatoes. Whole-grain, that is, unprocessed, forms have the most nutrients and fiber. For variety, try less familiar grain foods like polenta, couscous, millet, and quinoa.*

▶ *Eat at least five portions of fruits and vegetables each day. These can be chosen from a wide variety of fresh, frozen, and dried forms and include juices.*

▶ *Cut saturated fat, found mostly in meats and dairy products, to no more than 10 percent of your diet. By eating more fruits, vegetables, and whole-grain foods, it is easy to follow this third rule.*

EAT YOUR GREENS

The health benefits derived from eating plenty of fruits and vegetables can be seen by comparing dietary intake to rates of heart disease throughout western Europe.

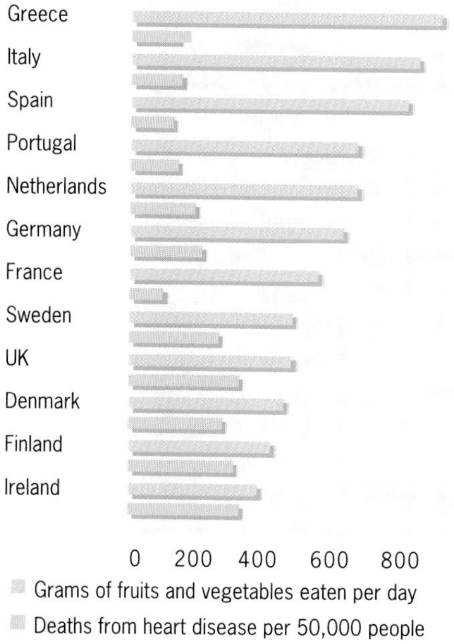

Greece
Italy
Spain
Portugal
Netherlands
Germany
France
Sweden
UK
Denmark
Finland
Ireland

0   200   400   600   800

■ Grams of fruits and vegetables eaten per day

■ Deaths from heart disease per 50,000 people

PREVENTING HEART DISEASE
Eating at least five portions of vegetables and fruits every day reduces the risk of heart disease by an estimated 20 percent.

the mid 19th century, our intake of refined carbohydrates has greatly increased.

Complex carbohydrates are composed of interlinked sugar molecules. Digestive enzymes break down these linked molecules into their constituent single sugars so that they can be absorbed into the bloodstream. Several hormones, in particular insulin, adrenaline, and glucagon, are involved in carbohydrate metabolism. These all work together to maintain a steady blood sugar (glucose) level. Glycogen stores are mobilized by adrenaline and glucagon, and it is these hormones that are directly responsible for raising blood sugar levels.

For glucose to be utilized by the body for energy, it has to cross from the blood into tissue cells, a process that requires insulin. Therefore, insulin lowers blood sugar by helping it to transfer into the cells where it is needed. In diabetics, who suffer from a shortage of insulin or an inability to fully utilize it, blood sugar levels become too high, but there is a corresponding shortage of glucose in the cells due to a shortage of usable insulin. The sufferer is left feeling weak and fatigued (see page 92).

PROTEIN

Proteins provide the building blocks of growth and tissue repair and are crucial also to the production of neurotransmitters—chemical messengers in the brain that convey signals important to such essential functions as memory, pleasure, alertness, and growth. They can also be converted into glycogen for energy.

Protein is made up of compounds called amino acids, of which there are 20. The body can produce 11 of them; the remaining 9 must be obtained from food. Animal foods provide all 9 of the essential amino acids; hence, they are called complete proteins. Except for soybeans (the closest to animal proteins), plants are missing or are low in one or more amino acids; to create a complete protein, a plant food low in one amino acid must be combined with one that is high in that compound. For example, beans, which are high in lysine and low in methionine, can be combined with grains, which are low in lysine and high in mehionine.

In a healthfully balanced diet protein should comprise 10 to 20 percent of daily caloric intake. The

drate not needed for immediate use will be stored in the liver and muscles as glycogen, and the liver will convert it back to glucose as needed. The body can store only enough glycogen to last for several hours of moderate activity. After that, more glucose has to be produced by converting protein (muscle) and then body fat stores.

The term carbohydrate refers to both the simple sugars and the starches, or complex carbohydrates. Simple sugars are the types found in fruits and products made with refined sucrose (table sugar). Starches are found in all grains, legumes, and starchy vegetables like potatoes and corn. Starches are the main sources of energy in most diets worldwide. (Nutritionists recommend that more than half of a healthy diet should consist of carbohydrates, at least 80 percent of which are starches.) Our ancestors ate considerably more complex carbohydrates than we in the Western world do today, and since

GLUCOSE
Every carbohydrate is broken down into monosaccharides, such as glucose (pictured below), which consists of a hexagonal molecular arrangement of carbon (blue), oxygen (orange), and hydrogen (yellow).

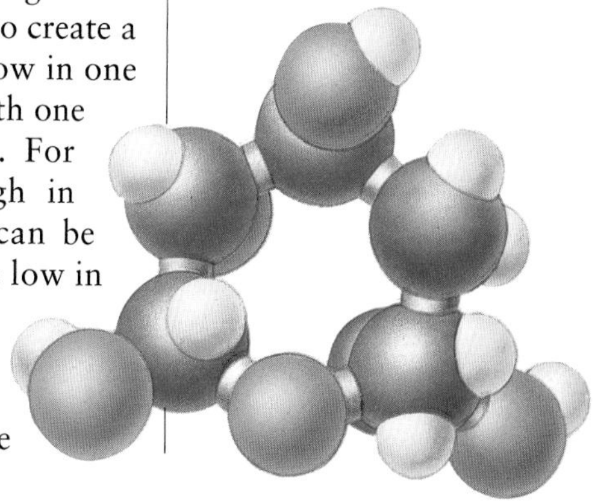

83

THE KREBS CYCLE AND ENERGY PRODUCTION

Inside each cell in the body reside a number of small energy factories called mitochondria. Within each of these a reaction takes place in which a chemical (ATP) splits and creates energy. By splitting, the chemical character of the ATP changes and it becomes ADP. The chemical is restored back to ATP with the use of fuel from glucose and other nutrients. It then splits again, repeating the cycle.

1 *The Krebs cycle is a complicated process in which glucose and other fuels combine to create phosphate molecules, which are the source of energy production.*

2 *A phosphate molecule from the Krebs cycle joins two phosphate molecules from adenosine diphosphate (ADP) to form energy-producing adenosine triphosphate (ATP).*

3 *The restored ATP splits, releasing energy and losing a phosphate molecule, thus becoming ADP. The process also uses oxygen and produces carbon dioxide as a by-product, which is then expelled from the lungs.*

Carbon dioxide

Krebs cycle produces phosphate

Glucose and other fuels

P Phosphate groups

ADP

ATP

Energy

ADP

4 *The ADP stays in this state until another phosphate molecule provided by the Krebs cycle becomes available.*

figure in North America tends to be much higher than this because so many people consume a lot of meat and dairy foods.

FAT

Fat serves as a storehouse for extra energy and also cushions many internal organs and provides insulation to keep the body temperature steady. Carbohydrates and proteins that are not needed for present use are stored as fat, or adipose tissue. When our weight remains steady, it's because we are making fat and using it up at equal rates.

In small amounts the fats in food are just as important to the body as carbohydrates and protein. They transport the fat-soluble vitamins A, D, E, and K and are essential to growth (in children), metabolism, and the manufacture of cell membranes and many hormones. They also make many foods palatable and provide a comfortably full feeling long after proteins and carbohydrates have been digested.

There are three types of dietary fats—saturated, monounsaturated, and polyunsaturated. Saturated fats, found mostly in meats and dairy products, become hard in cool temperatures and can stubbornly remain in arteries and the heart, causing poor heart and artery functioning. Monounsaturated and polyunsaturated fats are those that remain liquid in cool temperatures, such as vegetable and fish oils. There is evidence from the wide use of olive (monounsaturated) oil in the Mediterranean countries that these oils provide special benefits to health. Fish oils, which are high in the polyunsaturated omega-3 fatty acids, are particularly good for you. They not only are crucial for proper body functioning but also help lower levels of the type of cholesterol that clogs arteries. It has been suggested that you try to eat oily fish, such as tuna, salmon, and sardines, at least twice a week.

SUGAR

According to many food advertising campaigns, glucose and sucrose (table sugar) both help to maintain energy. This is true, but neither glucose nor sucrose is essential for a healthy diet because the body obtains glucose from the breakdown of complex carbohydrates, thus obtaining a gradual, continuous energy supply.

Excessive intake of refined sugar can result in hypoglycemia—low blood sugar levels (see pages 144–145). Foods high in refined sugar cause a rapid rise in blood

NUTRIENTS IN SOME COMMON FOODS

The table below lists a selection of common foods and their approximate nutritional components. When the fat content is followed by an asterisk, this indicates that a substantial proportion of the fat is saturated and the food should be eaten in moderation. (Saturated fat should be limited to 10 percent of daily calories.)

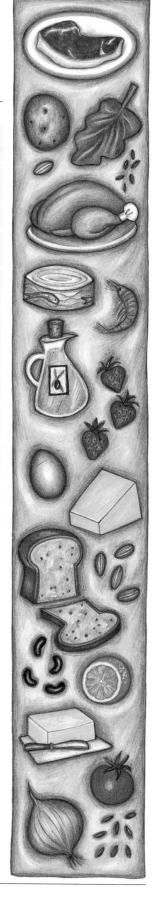

SOURCE	CALORIES	PROTEIN	CARB	FAT	VITAMINS	MINERALS
Chicken breast 85 g (3 oz)	130	24 g	0 g	3.0 g	B_2, B_3, B_6, B_{12}	Fe, K, P, S, Zn
Sirloin steak, broiled 85 g (3 oz)	176	27.4 g	0 g	6.0 g*	B_1, B_3, B_6, B_{12},	Fe, K, P, S, Zn
Ham, 85 g (3 oz)	155	15 g	3 g	9	B_2, B_3, B_6, B_{12}	Fe, K, Na, P, S, Zn
Egg, hard-cooked, 1 large	82	6.5 g	0.5 g	5.7 g	A, B_2, B_{12}, K	Ca, Fe, P, S, Zn
Salmon, broiled 85 g (3 oz)	179	16.7 g	0 g	7.4 g	A, B_3, B_6, B_{12}, D, E	Ca, F, I, K, P, S, Se, Zn
Shrimp, fried 85 g (3 oz)	192	17.4 g	8.4 g	9.3 g	B_3, B_{12}	Cu, F, Fe, I, K, Mg, Na, P, S, Zn
Olive oil, 1 tbsp	119	0 g	0 g	12.7 g		
Butter, 1 tbsp	102	0.1 g	0.1 g	10.4 g*	A	Na
Cheddar cheese, 25 g (1 oz)	113	7.1 g	0.6 g	8.3 g*	A, B_2, B_{12}, D	Ca, Na, P
Cottage cheese, 85 g (3 oz)	72	14.4 g	2.4 g	0.3 g	B_3	Na, P
Orange, 1 medium	71	1.1 g	18.1 g	0.3 g	A, B_1, C,	K, P
Strawberries, 8 large	55	1 g	12.5 g	0.7 g	C	Fe, K
Bread, whole-wheat 1 slice	168	7.2 g	33 g	2.1 g	B_1, B_3, B_6, E	Mg, Na, P, Zn
Brown rice, steamed 225 g (8 oz)	232	4.9 g	49.7 g	1.2 g	B_1, B_3, B_6, folic acid	Cu, Fe, K, Mg, Na, P, S, Zn
Almonds, shelled 55 g (2 oz)	340	10.6 g	11 g	29.2 g	B_1, B_2, B_3, folic acid	Ca, Cu, Fe, K, Mg, P, S, Zn
Kidney beans, cooked 225 g (8 oz)	218	14.4 g	39.6 g	0.9 g	B_1, folic acid	Cu, Fe, K, Mg, P, Zn
Potatoes, boiled 225 g (8 oz)	163	4.6 g	36.9 g	0.15 g	B_1, B_3, B_6, C,	Fe, K, Mg, P
Spinach, steamed 225 g (8 oz)	41	5.4 g	6.5 g	0.5 g	A, B_3, B_6, C, E, K, folic acid	Ca, Cu, Fe, K, Mg
Tomato, 1 medium	20	1 g	4.3 g	0.2 g	A, C, folic acid	K
Broccoli, 180 g (6 oz)	44	5 g	8 g	1 g	A, C, folic acid	Ca, Fe, K

Key to vitamins B_1 (Thiamine), B_2 (Riboflavin), B_3 (Niacin), B_6 (Pyridoxine)
Key to minerals Ca (Calcium), Cu (Copper), F (Fluorine), Fe (Iron), I (Iodine), K (Potassium), Mg (Magnesium), Na (Sodium), P (Phosphorus), S (Sulfur), Se (Selenium), Zn (Zinc)

sugar, which can lead to an excessive production of insulin, and blood sugar levels drop quickly, resulting in fatigue

The most successful treatment for this type of fatigue is to replace refined carbohydrates with complex carbohydrates eaten every three to four hours. Complex carbohydrates are digested more slowly, and the resulting glucose is released gradually into the bloodstream, giving a long-lasting supply. This reduces fatigue, lethargy, and dizziness, with the result that you have more energy throughout the day.

Energy swings

Swings in energy that are related to food can be modified by eating regularly—four to six small meals a day or three larger meals with small snacks in between—and basing more than half your diet on carbohydrates, at least 80 percent of them complex. Some nutritional supplements (see pages 94–110) may help in the control of blood sugar. These should be taken only with the guidance of a doctor or dietitian and used in combination with appropriate dietary measures.

SUPPLEMENTS THAT CAN HELP BOOST ENERGY

A sensible and varied diet usually provides all the vitamins and minerals that the average person needs. Supplementing a diet with vitamins and/or minerals may be necessary, however, for certain people Among them are pregnant and nursing women, bottle-fed infants, elderly people, dieters, alcoholics, and cancer patients. Taking megadoses of supplements—many times the American Recommended Dietary Allowance (RDA) or Canadian Recommended Nutrient Intake (RNI)—without medical guidance is not advised.

SUPPLEMENT	BENEFITS AND FUNCTIONS	TARGET GROUPS	RDA AND RNI
Vitamin A	Needed for growth and healthy skin, hair, eyes.	Children, smokers	2,600–3,300 I.U.
Vitamin B complex	Releases energy; promotes healthy skin and nerves; aids production of hormones and antibodies.	Pregnant or breastfeeding mothers, those suffering emotional stress	As directed
Vitamin C	Is needed for healthy tissues and wound healing; fights infection; helps absorb iron.	Pregnant or breastfeeding mothers, the elderly, convalescents, drinkers and smokers	60 mg (RDA) 30–40 mg (RNI)
Folic acid	Is important for the production of red blood cells, DNA, RNA, and synthesis of amino acids.	Women planning pregnancy or who are in early pregnancy need twice the RDA or RNI.	180–200 mcg (RDA) 180–230 mcg (RNI)
Vitamin E	Maintains red blood cells and muscles; reduces damaging effects of oxidation.	Women taking the contraceptive pill or hormone replacement treatments	8–10 mg (RDA) 10–15 I.U. (RNI)
Iron	Is essential for development of red blood cells.	Menstruating women, vegetarians	9–15 mg
Magnesium	Stimulates bone growth and muscle movement.	Heavy drinkers and people with poor diets	200–350 mg
Selenium	Protects against damage from free radicals.	The elderly, breastfeeding women, dieters	55–70 mcg (RDA)
Zinc	Is needed for enzyme production, immune function, and normal growth	The elderly and anyone with a poor or restricted diet	12–15 mg (RDA) 9–12 mg (RNI)
Coenzyme Q10	Increases release of energy from food.	The elderly, athletes, people with poor diets	None
Garlic	Is good for the heart and immune system.	Everyone	None
Gingko biloba	Maintains blood circulation; ncreases blood to the brain.	People suffering from poor circulation or poor memory and ability to concentrate	None
Ginseng	Helps maintain the natural balance of body systems.	The elderly, athletes, stressed people	None
Gamma linoleic acid (GLA)	Helps body functions to run smoothly and improves the skin.	Premenstrual women with tender breasts	None
Omega-3 fatty acids	Maintains healthy membranes and transports fats around the body.	People suffering from arthritis, rheumatism, or poor circulation	None

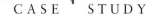

A Constantly Tired Woman

The root of many energy problems lies in a diet that lacks some vital nutrients, which prevents a body from functioning as well as it should and interrupts the natural course of energy production. With the help of a dietitian, such deficiencies can be corrected through dietary changes and supplements to achieve the right balance of nutrients.

Kate is a 32-year-old divorcee with a 7-year-old son. She used to work full-time as a legal secretary, but a year ago she started getting frequent headaches and feeling constantly tired, and she cut back her work to part-time. She attributed her fatigue to the strain of dealing with her ex-husband and bringing up her son on her own.

Kate was also suffering from PMS, which made her feel weak just before her period. Her diet consisted mainly of toast for breakfast, a doughnut for a midmorning snack, a sandwich for lunch, and a frozen dinner in the evening. She was also drinking six cups of coffee a day. Kate's doctor found she was fine physically, except for being slightly anemic, and referred her to a dietitian.

WHAT SHOULD KATE DO?

Kate needs to have regular meals and snacks based largely on complex carbohydrates to keep her blood sugar up and prevent the shaky feelings and headaches. Her whole diet needs to be lower in fat and sugar and higher in iron-rich foods and fiber. Kate should also cut down on caffeine to help relieve the symptoms of PMS and encourage restful sleep. If she eats at least five helpings of fruits and vegetables a day, these will provide her with the important vitamins, minerals, and fiber she needs. Including soy products like tofu in her diet may also ease PMS symptoms because the phytoestrogens in soy decrease the effects of high estrogen levels that are common in PMS.

DIET
Habitually eating processed foods that have little nutritional value can reduce your energy levels in the long run.

EATING HABITS
Irregular meals and snacks that are high in sugar encourage energy peaks and troughs, leaving you drained and tired.

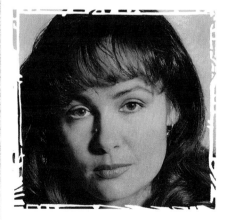

EMOTIONAL STRESS
Letting other people's demands get you down can drain your emotional energy.

Action Plan

DIET
Eat more iron-rich foods, such as lean meat, fish, and beans, plus citrus fruits, high in vitamin C, for iron absorption. Cut back on refined foods, salt, and caffeine.

EATING HABITS
Cook in the evening with fresh ingredients instead of defrosting a processed meal. Snack on whole-wheat crackers, cheese, and fruit.

EMOTIONAL STRESS
Try to resolve old disputes that are draining energy. Exercise regularly, both to relieve stress and to build up energy levels.

HOW THINGS TURNED OUT FOR KATE

The dietitian recommended a diet that included lots of fruits, vegetables, and whole grains, modest amounts of meat, and little sugar. It was difficult at first—especially cutting down on coffee and sweets and doing more cooking—but within a few weeks Kate had more energy. She now takes her son swimming every week and is looking for a full-time job. She also discussed her marriage problems with a counselor and feels more in control of her life.

ENERGY LEVELS THROUGHOUT THE DAY

Eating meals and snacks that keep pace with your energy needs will help maintain your alertness and feeling of well-being at steady levels all day long.

STAYING ALERT
The key to all-day energy is to replenish your fuel reserves every few hours with meals or snacks containing high-fiber complex carbohydrates and/or protein. These are absorbed slowly into the system, releasing energy at a steady rate over a long period of time.

Scientists have found that not only what you eat and drink but when can affect how tired or alert you are throughout the day. However, the body plays a big part too, as it has its own natural cycles, known as circadian rhythms. Circadian rhythms take you through a constant series of peaks and troughs over 24 hours. Usually there are two big dips in alertness: one late at night and a smaller one after lunch at around 2 P.M. Certain foods and beverages can exacerbate the low points. For example, the larger the meal at lunchtime, the bigger the post-lunch dip, especially if lunch includes alcohol. Many cultures make use of this natural after-lunch dip by providing time in the middle of the day for a nap.

Some studies have shown that eating a high-protein lunch at midday and a high-carbohydrate, low-fat meal in the early evening is the best way to maintain alert-ness. But other research has failed to sup-port this idea, and it remains controversial. (You can try this approach to see if it works for you. Differences in metabolism seem to have some impact on the results.)

Some research is being focused on a hor-mone called cholecystokinin, released by the gut when food is eaten, especially fatty food. Early indications are that this hor-mone makes the research subjects feel more sluggish and inert.

THE IMPORTANCE OF BREAKFAST

Breakfast is a crucial meal because it follows the long overnight fast. Studies have shown that eating breakfast improves cognitive function by causing short-term metabolic and hormonal changes. These occur follow-ing the supply of energy and nutrients to the brain. A number of research studies have shown breakfast to be of particular impor-

Breakfast of whole-wheat cereal, milk, and fruit juice kick-starts the body and mind into action. Eggs are also good for supplying energy throughout the morning.

A midmorning snack of fruit, like a banana or apple, provides a boost in carbohydrate levels.

A protein-rich lunch that includes meat, fish, beans, cheese, or eggs, accompanied by fruit or salad, fuels you for the afternoon.

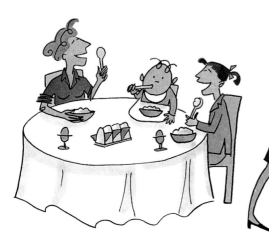

DIET AND NEUROCHEMICALS

Scientists have found links between daily fluctuations in a substance called serotonin and the consumption of carbohydrate-rich foods. Serotonin is a hormone found in tissues, blood, and, more important, in nerves, where it acts as a neurotransmitter—a chemical messenger that induces sleepiness and elevates mood and relaxation. Research has found that following the ingestion of a meal high in carbohydrates, there is an increase in the rate at which the brain produces serotonin. This is thought to happen because serotonin is made from the amino acid tryptophan, which is provided in protein foods along with other amino acids. Tryptophan needs to compete with all the other amino acids for the same entry points into the brain and is therefore in limited supply. However, foods high in carbohydrates stimulate the release of insulin, which has the effect of pushing all the other amino acids into the muscle cells and thus allowing the free passage of tryptophan into the brain. Therefore, carbohydrate-rich foods can enhance your mood and improve your sleep.

If you do not eat breakfast, there will be rapid changes in your metabolism; for example, blood glucose levels will decline, and this can trigger a stress response, which interferes with concentration. If such an effect occurs regularly, it can, for example, undermine a child's progress at school. Several studies have examined the link between brain function and breakfast in schoolchildren; skipping breakfast seems particularly to affect the speed and accuracy of information retrieval in the working memory. In Canada and the United States, a number of schools have established breakfast programs for children from low-income families to help alleviate this problem.

DIET FOR SLEEP PROBLEMS

Sleep can be enhanced by eating a light carbohydrate snack just before going to bed. Carbohydrate increases serotonin production in the brain (see box, left) and also prevents you from feeling hungry during the night. In addition, drawing blood away from the brain to the stomach encourages sleepiness. However, you should avoid heavy meals late in the evening. Circadian rhythm experts in Liverpool have found that people who regularly eat late at night are susceptible to digestive disorders and stomach ulcers. Also, the body has trouble entering deep sleep when it is in the first stages of food digestion, and the result is fatigue and impaired body functioning. Deficiencies in copper, magnesium, and the B vitamins may also interfere with sleep.

tance in people who are nutritionally at risk, especially children and the elderly.

SOURCES OF COMPLEX CARBOHYDRATES

Complex carbohydrates, or starches, are found in all plant foods but are especially high in grains and legumes. The following foods are good sources of them:

▶ *Bread*
▶ *Breakfast cereals*
▶ *Corn*
▶ *Crackers*
▶ *Pasta*
▶ *Potatoes*
▶ *Rice*
▶ *Beans, peas, lentils*

A midafternoon snack of milk or yogurt, fresh fruit, or vegetable juice will help revive sinking energy levels.

A dinner based on a starch, such as pasta or potatoes, and lightly cooked vegetables will help to replenish the energy used during the day.

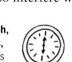

A light snack of complex carbohydrates before bed, such as a few crackers or a slice of whole-grain toast, will help you sleep more soundly.

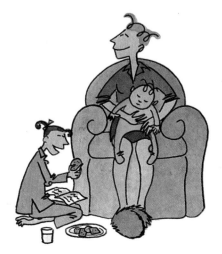

ENERGY LEVELS AND SPECIAL DIETS

If you are following a restricted diet, you may face challenges in maintaining high energy levels. Recognizing the problem areas can help you balance your diet and stay healthy.

Many people are on special diets, either by choice or by necessity. Some willingly give up animal products for philosophical reasons; others have to restrict their diets because of health problems such as diabetes, arthritis, kidney stones, allergies, or food intolerances.

VEGETARIANISM

Vegetarianianism has become increasingly popular. There is some concern about the nutritional adequacy of plant-based diets, but with careful planning, most are consistent with good nutrition and can even provide a number of health benefits (see box, opposite).

Of the several types of vegetarian diets, the most common is ovolacto, whose practitioners omit meat but include milk, other dairy products, and eggs, as well as plant foods; lactovegetarians also exclude eggs. Vegans eliminate completely all foods that come from animals; some even exclude honey. A vegan diet is based entirely on cereals and cereal products, vegetables, nuts, fruits, legumes, and seeds.

Nutrients in vegetarian diets

Because most plant foods contain more water and fiber and less fat than foods of animal origin, vegetarian diets usually have fewer calories than conventional ones, and this can help adults to maintain an ideal weight. But for growing children or anyone who has a poor appetite, very restrictive vegetarian plans can pose the risk of not getting enough energy. There have been incidences of malnutrition and retarded growth in children raised on very limited plant-based diets. Vegetarian parents should consult a nutritionist or dietitian for advice about their children's nutritional needs.

There is also concern about sufficient protein in a vegetarian diet. The minimum protein recommendation for an adult is 10 percent of daily energy intake, or 50 grams a day in a diet of 2,000 calories. This is met easily by a diet of mixed plant and animal proteins. The daily goal for vegans, however, should be 25 percent higher—or 63 grams a day in a 2,000-calorie diet.

Vegetarians must be careful to combine plant proteins so that they complement each other and provide complete proteins equivalent to those in animal foods. (Soy products are useful because soy is the only plant source of complete protein.) The rule is to combine legumes with grains, seeds, or nuts. Some examples are rice and lentils, peanut butter and bread, chickpeas and sesame seeds, and pasta and kidney beans. For those

---

COSMIC ENERGY FORCES: *The Moon*

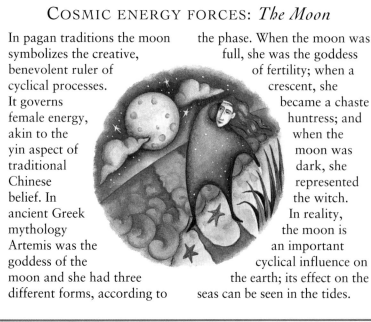

In pagan traditions the moon symbolizes the creative, benevolent ruler of cyclical processes. It governs female energy, akin to the yin aspect of traditional Chinese belief. In ancient Greek mythology Artemis was the goddess of the moon and she had three different forms, according to the phase. When the moon was full, she was the goddess of fertility; when a crescent, she became a chaste huntress; and when the moon was dark, she represented the witch. In reality, the moon is an important cyclical influence on the earth; its effect on the seas can be seen in the tides.

vegetarians who eat dairy products, a little added milk or cheese will enhance the plant protein of any dish.

Vegetarian diets and vitamins

Studies have shown that vegetarians usually have higher intakes of most vitamins than typical meat eaters. Vegans, however, can be deficient in three vitamins: D, B_2, and B_{12}.

Vitamin D may be a problem because the main sources are of animal origin—eggs, oily fish, liver—or it is added to milk products that are fortified. The vitamin can be made in skin exposed to sunlight, however, so vegans who spend plenty of time outside should not be deficient.

Vitamin B_{12} is produced by bacteria, fungi, and algae, and it accumulates only in animals, so a diet based on plants alone tends to be deficient in B_{12}. Recent research has found that many plant-based foods previously thought to contain B_{12} do not, so consuming B_{12}-fortified foods is advisable.

The major sources of riboflavin (vitamin B_2) are dairy products and meat, and so the dietary intake of this vitamin can be low for vegans. Several studies have shown no major health problems as a result, possibly because many cereals are enriched with it.

HEALTH BENEFITS OF VEGETARIAN DIETS

A vegetarian diet offers many health benefits because it is lower in fat, especially saturated fat, and higher in complex carbohydrates and fiber than conventional diets. Studies have shown that vegetarians on average have lower weight and blood fats, lower rates of heart disease, strokes, and certain cancers, and fewer intestinal disorders, such as constipation and diverticulosis. In addition, vegetarian diets have been used successfully to help reduce blood cholesterol and manage angina, hypertension, and obesity, even asthma and rheumatoid arthritis. Vegetarians may also benefit from the avoidance of animal-related diseases and food poisoning, which have been problems in recent years.

DIABETES

Diabetes mellitus is a chronic metabolic disease in which the body does not produce or does not fully utilize insulin (see page 142) and therefore cannot properly metabolize

ENERGY-RICH FOOD FOR VEGETARIANS

It is crucial that those on vegetarian diets pay special attention to their energy levels. The following foods contain many of the nutrients that vegetarians need.

▶ *Nuts and nut spreads*
▶ *Dried beans, peas, and other legumes*
▶ *Dried fruits*
▶ *Tofu, soy milk, and other soy products*
▶ *Vegetable oils*
▶ *For the ovolacto vegetarian: eggs and milk and other dairy products*

MINERALS AND THE VEGETARIAN DIET

Some minerals that are abundant in animal foods are available in plants in lesser amounts (calcium and zinc) or less easily absorbed forms (iron). Others are contained primarily in the bran or germ of cereals, so these are best eaten in their whole-grain rather than refined forms. Accompanying iron-rich plants like beans and spinach with foods high in vitamin C enhances absorption of their iron.

HEALTHY CHOICES
Each of these high-protein foods, in the quantities shown, provides 50–100 mg of calcium, 1 mg of zinc, and 2 mg of iron (except soybeans, which have 4 mg). The beans are given in cooked weights.

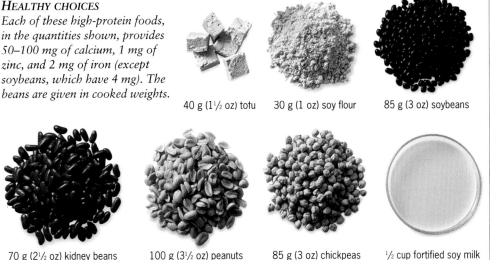

40 g (1½ oz) tofu   30 g (1 oz) soy flour   85 g (3 oz) soybeans

70 g (2½ oz) kidney beans   100 g (3½ oz) peanuts   85 g (3 oz) chickpeas   ½ cup fortified soy milk

DIETARY NEEDS OF THE UNDERWEIGHT

People who are underweight (15 percent or more below the low end of the range for height and age) lack energy reserves and are vulnerable to illness. To gain weight healthfully, increase food intake gradually, adding 500 to 750 extra calories a day, and select foods that are higher in calories; for example, eat avocados instead of cucumbers. Also, avoid caffeine, which suppresses appetite.

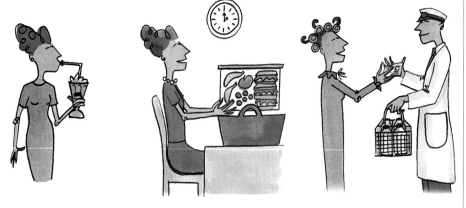

Eat high-calorie and nutritious snacks, including roasted nuts and seeds, dried fruits, and milk shakes. Avoid sugary foods.

Eat regularly and never miss a meal. This will keep your energy levels steady and build up your nutrient levels and energy stores.

Have whole-milk dairy products, such as regular milk and cheese, rather than skim milk. These are high in protein as well as fat.

carbohydrates. Glucose builds up in the blood, but the brain and other tissues that need it are unable to utilize it. There are two forms: type I, or insulin-dependent diabetes (IDD), in which the body stops producing insulin, and type II, or non-insulin-dependent diabetes (NIDD), in which the body produces inadequate insulin or is unable to use it fully. Type I is treated with insulin injections; type II is controlled through diet, drugs, and exercise.

Type I diabetes often strikes people when they are young, whereas type II appears most often in middle age. One early sign of diabetes is unexplained fatigue. Increased thirst, urination, and irritability are also common. About half of type II diabetics go undiagnosed, however, because they exhibit no symptoms.

The aim of dietary treatment is to stop the harmful effects of diabetes by keeping blood glucose levels as close to normal as possible. Diabetics should generally have meals that are a mixture of proteins, fats, and carbohydrates, with high-fiber complex carbohydrates making up the bulk. Because age, weight, and other medical conditions can affect nutritional needs, a dietitian should be consulted for specific meal plans. (Dietary measures for diabetes are covered more fully on page 143.)

It has been estimated that 75 to 80 percent of NIDD sufferers are overweight. For these people the caloric content of the diet has probably the greatest effect on long-term diabetic control. Research has shown that losing weight makes it easier to control the disease with diet and exercise alone.

CHROMIUM DEFICIENCY AND DIABETES

Chromium regulates the action and efficiency of insulin in the body. A number of studies conducted in the United States in the 1990s found that the body's chromium decreases with age, especially in men. This suggests that some of the diseases associated with aging, such as non-insulin-dependent diabetes and heart disease, may be linked to age-related decreases in chromium levels. Chromium is found in liver, cheese, nuts, and whole-grain cereals; a diet high in refined carbohydrates could result in chromium deficiency. Chromium supplements have been shown to improve insulin control in diabetics.

ENERGY BOOST

Broccoli is one of the most nutrient-rich vegetables and is surprisingly high in protein. Other nutrients include vitamins C, B$_2$, and folic acid.

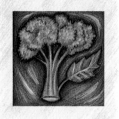

Losing Weight

A weight-loss plan can be a tremendous strain if you love food. However, many people also suffer from a fundamental loss of energy with a decrease in calorie intake. This can be remedied by a high-carbohydrate, low-fat diet plan.

The key to any diet is to reduce the intake of fuel and increase the amount of exercise so that you use up the reserves that you have stored as fat in your body. The best way to do this without compromising your health and energy levels is by adopting a high-nutrient, low-fat, low-sugar diet that will keep you satisfied and healthy without so many calories. Low-calorie alternatives to many foods are now widely available, allowing you to eat the same foods with lower energy values. However, to keep your energy levels high, you need to include plenty of fiber and complex carbohydrates in your diet to help you to get through the day without your blood sugar levels falling too low and your stomach rumbling.

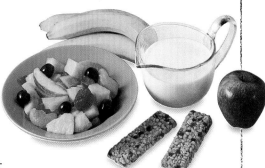

KEEPING YOUR ENERGY LEVELS HIGH
Eating snacks throughout the day will help to keep hunger pangs at bay and energy levels high. However, you must make sure that your food choices are low in fat and high in nutrients.

CHOOSING LOW-FAT, LOW-SUGAR, HIGH-CARBOHYDRATE ALTERNATIVES

Complex carbohydrates are absorbed slowly, maintaining a stream of nutrients and energy pouring into your system over an extended period of time and preventing you from feeling hungry or lacking in energy. These should be selected over sugary foods, which may give you instant energy boosts but will tire you in the long term, and fatty foods, which are high in calories. Healthier alternatives are described below.

SUBSTITUTE	INSTEAD OF	WHY MAKE THE CHANGE?
Skim or low-fat milk; low-fat or nonfat cheese, yogurt, and sour cream	Whole-milk products; cream; regular sour cream	Because of its calcium, milk is an important part of a normal diet. however, milk fat is high in calories and saturated fat.
Low-fat cereal bar	Candy bar	Cereals provide complex carbohydrates that release energy gradually.
Fruit juice	Soft drinks	Soft drinks have empty calories; their sugar unbalances blood sugar levels.
Low-calorie dessert	Cake, cookies, pastry	Helps control weight and health while still satisfying a sweet tooth.
Trimmed or extra-lean meat	Fatty meat	Much of the fat in meat is saturated and bad for the heart and arteries.
Bran or whole-grain cereal	Cornflakes	Increasing the fiber in your diet aids regularity and fills you up without adding extra calories.
Steamed, broiled, or poached foods	Fried foods	Frying food increases nutrient loss and adds needless calories.
Nonfat mayonnaise and salad dressing	Regular mayonnaise	Calories are cut without sacrificing flavor.
Fruit salad	Cake or cookies	Fruit provides more nutrients and fewer calories.
Baked or boiled potatoes	French-fried potatoes	French fries are very high in fat.
Low-calorie sauce	Regular sauce	Sauces are often misleadingly high in fat and calories.
Fresh or dried fruit	Potato or corn chips	Fruit provides fewer calories and more nutrients.

THE ENERGY NUTRIENTS

Requirements for various nutrients vary slightly from person to person and depend on many factors, including age, height and weight, gender, physical condition, and lifestyle.

The human body needs a range of vitamins and minerals in just the right balance to keep it operating efficiently, but some nutrients are of greater importance to energy production than others; these "energy" nutrients are described in the pages that follow. Understanding how each nutrient works within the body and the effects that even mild deficiencies can have on your vitality should help you determine if any fatigue you are experiencing could be caused by a nutritional deficiency. (However, suspicion of a deficiency should not lead you to take supplements that exceed recommended daily intakes without the advice of a doctor or nutritionist.)

A brief description is given of how each nutrient works in the body and the principal foods in which each it can be found. Some of the best food sources for each nutrient are illustrated as well. The recommended dietary requirements, if any, are given in either milligrams (mg) or micrograms (mcg). Recipes suggest how to increase each of the nutrients in your diet in easy and pleasing ways. After all, eating healthfully does not have to mean depriving yourself of flavor and the enjoyment of food.

A large and growing body of research is being amassed that shows the links between nutrient deficiencies and a lack of energy. Magnesium supplements, for example, have been found to significantly alleviate fatigue problems in people who are slightly deficient in this mineral. The B vitamins have been widely recognized by medical experts for their beneficial contribution to metabolism and psychological health, both of which, when improved, raise energy levels. Advances in our understanding of neurotransmitters have led medical researchers to harness amino acids such as carnitine for their energy-boosting qualities. Coenzyme Q10 has also generated great interest since it was discovered to improve metabolism substantially. New and exciting links between energy and micronutrients are emerging in research centers throughout the world, and more are expected in the future.

THE STRUCTURE OF VITAMINS

All vitamins have complex molecular structures that consist mainly of the elements carbon, oxygen, nitrogen, and hydrogen. Their structures allow them to form bonds with other molecules within food. With cooking, many of the bonds weaken, allowing the vitamins to drain out.

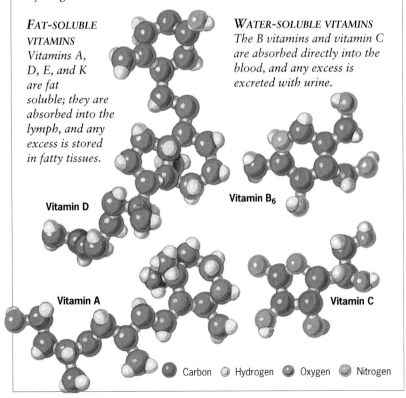

FAT-SOLUBLE VITAMINS
Vitamins A, D, E, and K are fat soluble; they are absorbed into the lymph, and any excess is stored in fatty tissues.

WATER-SOLUBLE VITAMINS
The B vitamins and vitamin C are absorbed directly into the blood, and any excess is excreted with urine.

Vitamin D

Vitamin B₆

Vitamin A

Vitamin C

● Carbon ● Hydrogen ● Oxygen ● Nitrogen

HOW YOUR BODY USES VITAMINS AND MINERALS

Although most vitamins and minerals are required throughout the body for general functions, many play a specific role—or a number of roles—in enabling particular systems to function properly. When one system or body part functions poorly as a result of deficiency in a nutrient, it can affect the entire body. The interaction between minerals and vitamins is so complex that a deficiency or excess of one is likely to lead to other problems. All of the following vitamins and minerals can be obtained through the diet. However, vitamin D can also be synthesized in the body when the skin is exposed to sunlight, and vitamin K can be produced by bacteria in the intestinal tract.

Skin and hair need vitamins A, B$_2$, B$_3$, B$_6$, and B$_{12}$, biotin, sulfur, and zinc. Healthy eyes and eyesight benefit from vitamin A and zinc. Healthy teeth need vitamins C and D, calcium, phosphorus, fluorine, and magnesium.

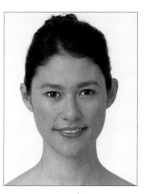

Nervous system functioning can be strengthened by these nutrients: vitamins B$_1$, B$_6$, B$_{12}$, biotin, and E, plus calcium, potassium, sodium, and magnesium.

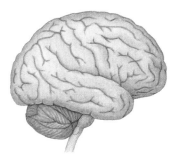

Energy production can be improved by vitamins B$_1$, B$_2$, B$_3$, B$_5$, biotin, calcium, chromium, copper, iodine, iron, magnesium, phosphorus, and potassium. Proper muscle functioning depends on vitamin B$_1$, calcium, magnesium, potassium, and sodium.

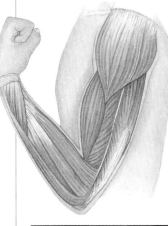

Cardiovascular strength is a crucial constituent of good health. Important nutrients include vitamin B$_1$, calcium, copper, magnesium, sodium, potassium, and selenium.

Healthy blood cell formation is assisted by vitamins B$_6$, B$_{12}$, E, folic acid, copper, and iron. Blood clotting depends on vitamin K and calcium.

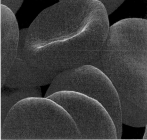

VITAL BALANCE The correct balance of minerals and vitamins is needed to ensure proper body functioning. A healthfully balanced diet should provide you with your daily needs.

Healthy bones need vitamins A, C, and D, calcium, copper, fluorine, phosphorus, and magnesium. Babies and children need more of these nutrients for healthy growth.

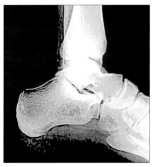

▼▼

Thiamine

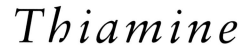

Thiamine, also known as vitamin B$_1$, plays a crucial role in converting carbohydrates, proteins, and fats into energy and preventing the buildup of toxins that are natural by-products of metabolism in the body.

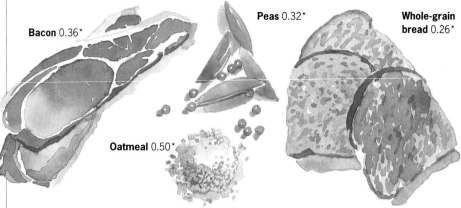

Bacon 0.36*

Peas 0.32*

Whole-grain bread 0.26*

Oatmeal 0.50*

*mg per 100 g

THE DISCOVERY OF THIAMINE

Beriberi—a degenerative disease of the nerves and heart caused by a severe deficiency of thiamine—was first noted in 1873 by a Dutch naval doctor. In the 1890s, Christiaan Eijkman, a physician in the Dutch East Indies, found that beriberi could be cured by adding the polishings of rice (the part removed during processing) to the diet. In 1911 biochemist Casimir Funk, working at the Lister Institute in London, isolated what he termed a "vitamine" that prevented beriberi. However, what he had actually discovered was niacin. It was two Dutch scientists working in Java who finally identified thiamine, or vitamin B$_1$, in 1926.

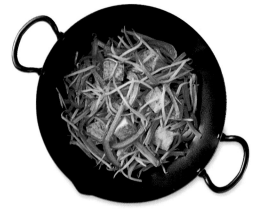

TOFU WITH CHINESE VEGETABLES
Slice a green onion and green pepper and julienne a carrot; stir-fry in a hot pan for a few minutes. Add diced firm tofu and stir-fry 5 minutes more. Add a few hand-fuls of mung bean sprouts and a splash of soy sauce and cook briefly until the bean sprouts are slightly soft. Tofu and other soy products are rich in thiamine.

Thiamine is crucial to the body's energy production. The amount of thiamine needed is partly related to the quantity and type of foods consumed. Carbohydrates require more thiamine to metabolize them than fat does. There are also a number of naturally occurring substances that prevent absorption of thiamine; they are found in coffee, tea, and certain fruits and vegetables, including spinach and cabbage, also in raw fish and shellfish. The heat of cooking destroys thiamine, and it is leached by cooking water.

In underdeveloped countries severe thiamine deficiency, known as beriberi—Sinhalese for "extreme weakness"—is usually the result of diets based largely on white rice and/or raw fish. In developed countries alcoholism is the main cause of deficiency, and usually several other nutrients are lacking as well.

Mild thiamine deficiency causes fatigue, listlessness, irritability, mood swings, digestive problems, numbness in the legs, and retarded growth in children. A severe lack of this

SOURCES AND REQUIREMENTS

Sources
Particularly good sources include whole grains, pork, beef, legumes, brewer's yeast, brown rice, and soy products. Refined grains, such as white rice and white flour, have substantially reduced levels unless they have been enriched.

Dietary requirements
Requirements in the U.S. are 1.2–1.3 mg for men, 1–1.1 mg for women; in Canada the figures are 0.8–1.3 mg for men; 0.8–0.9 for women. The needs for pregnant and nursing women are half again as much.

vitamin can lead to rapid deterioration in both the heart and muscle function and inflammation or degeneration of the nerves. Thiamine deficiency may also be a contributing factor in such nonspecific conditions as weight loss and depression.

▲▲

Riboflavin

Riboflavin, also known as vitamin B_2, plays a major role in the release of energy from carbohydrates, proteins, and fats; aids in adrenal function; and helps maintain tissues in the skin and eyes.

Riboflavin, discovered in the 1930s when it was isolated from yeast extract, plays a major role in the formation of a number of enzymes. These enzymes help with the removal of hydrogen molecules and the introduction of oxygen molecules. During this process certain essential substances are metabolized and energy is released. Riboflavin is crucial in the metabolism of carbohydrates, proteins, and fats, as well as in the oxidation of several other substances. It is also neces-

sary to the metabolism of vitamins B_3, B_6, and folic acid. (This is the reason that some people with riboflavin deficiency have symptoms of vitamin B_6 deficiency.)

Because riboflavin is water soluble, it is easily lost in the cooking water for vegetables. It is also removed in the milling of grains, though it is usually added back to enriched flours.

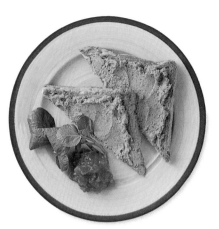

CHICKEN LIVER PATÉ ON WHOLE-WHEAT TOAST
This simple repast can be eaten as a nutritious snack, an appetizer, or a light meal. You can buy the pâté ready-made or prepare your own. Liver is one of the best sources of riboflavin and a number of other nutrients as well.

SYMPTOMS OF DEFICIENCY

Early symptoms include sore and burning lips and tongue. These can also occur with vitamin B_6 deficiency, but dryness, cracking, and peeling of the lips is a particular characteristic of insufficient riboflavin. The skin on the face becomes red, oily, and scaly, especially at the sides of the nose. Also, unlike vitamin B_6 shortage, there may be a sensitivity to light and other eye irritations. Some people with riboflavin deficiency complain also of burning feet.

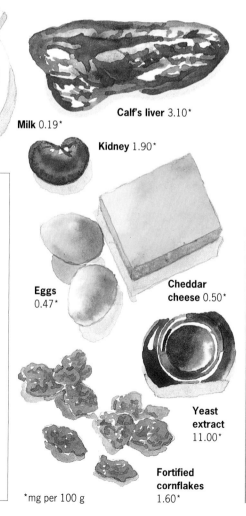

Milk 0.19*

Calf's liver 3.10*

Kidney 1.90*

Eggs 0.47*

Cheddar cheese 0.50*

Yeast extract 11.00*

Fortified cornflakes 1.60*

*mg per 100 g

SOURCES AND REQUIREMENTS

Sources
Major food sources of riboflavin include dairy products, yeast extract, whole-grain and enriched cereal products, meat (especially organs), and dark green leafy vegetables, including spinach and broccoli. Riboflavin is fairly stable when heated, particularly with dry heat (as in an oven), but it deteriorates quickly on exposure to light, especially sunlight.

Dietary requirements
The RDAs in the U.S. are 1.4–1.7 mg for adult men, 1.2–1.3 mg for women. The RNIs in Canada are 1.3 mg for men, 1.1 mg for women. Pregnant and nursing women require 0.3—0.5 mg more.

Niacin

Niacin, sometimes called vitamin B₃, is crucial to the formation of certain enzymes involved in metabolism of carbohydrates, proteins, and fats to produce energy. It also enhances the health of the skin and nerves.

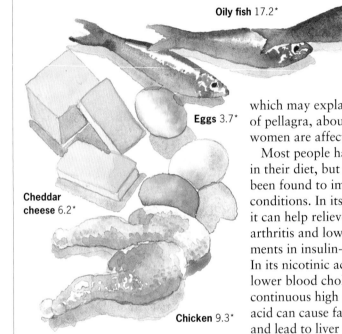

Oily fish 17.2*

Eggs 3.7*

Cheddar cheese 6.2*

Chicken 9.3*

*mg niacin equivalent per 100 g

which may explain why in epidemics of pellagra, about twice as many women are affected as men.

Most people have sufficient niacin in their diet, but supplements have been found to improve some medical conditions. In its niacinamide form, it can help relieve the stiffness of arthritis and lower insulin requirements in insulin-dependent diabetes. In its nicotinic acid form it can help lower blood cholesterol levels. But continuous high doses of nicotinic acid can cause fatigue and hot flushes and lead to liver disorders, peptic ulcers, and elevated blood sugar levels.

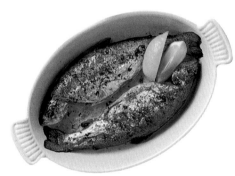

BAKED TROUT WITH LEMON
Blend juice of one lemon with 2 tbsp olive oil and crushed garlic. Spoon the mixture over the fish; bake in a 350°F oven for 20 minutes, turning halfway through the cooking. Serve with lemon wedges and a mixed green salad. Oily fish, such as trout, tuna, sardines, and cod, are all excellent sources of niacin.

There are two main forms of niacin, nicotinic acid and niacinamide, also called nicotinamide. Symptoms of mild deficiency include mouth sores and diarrhea. Severe deficiency produces a condition known as pellagra, which has three major and chronic symptoms—dermatitis, diarrhea, and dementia. If untreated, it can result in death.

Niacin can be synthesized from the amino acid tryptophan (see page 107). It takes 60 mg of tryptophan to provide 1 mg of niacin. Many foods are therefore described in terms of their "niacin equivalent" (NE), which is dependent on the content of both niacin and tryptophan. The conversion of tryptophan into niacin is hindered by estrogen,

SOURCES AND REQUIREMENTS

Sources
Major food sources include seafood, lean meat, poultry, milk, legumes, eggs, whole grains, and enriched cereals. White mushrooms contain modest amounts.

Dietary requirements
An average intake of about 19 mg per day of niacin equivalent for men and 15 mg a day for women is recommended in the United States. In Canada the recommendation for both men and women is 7.2 mg for every 1,000 calories consumed.

Pantothenic acid

Like the other B vitamins, pantothenic acid, also known as vitamin B₅, plays a major role in energy production and is required for the metabolism of carbohydrates, fats, and proteins.

Pantothenic acid is important not only for the metabolism of carbohydrates, fats, and proteins but also for the production of cholesterol and the proper functioning of the adrenal hormones. Because this vitamin is found to some degree in most foods, no known cases of deficiency have been documented. However, supplements are sometimes recommended for people who are under chronic stress or suffer from arthritis.

Experimental studies in which a deficiency of pantothenic acid was produced found that signs of deficiency take several weeks to appear. Observations of intake and excretion suggest that the body has considerable stores, which can be drawn upon in times of a dietary deficiency. The symptoms of deficiency include fatigue, headaches, weakness, impaired muscle coordination, and muscle cramps.

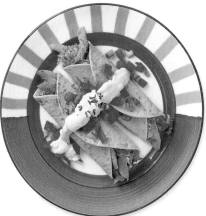

SPICY CHICKEN TORTILLAS
Stir-fry strips of chicken breast in a little olive oil, adding the juice of a lime at the end. Roll up in tortillas along with shredded lettuce. Add salsa and sour cream to taste. All these ingredients except the oil provide pantothenic acid.

*mg per 100 g

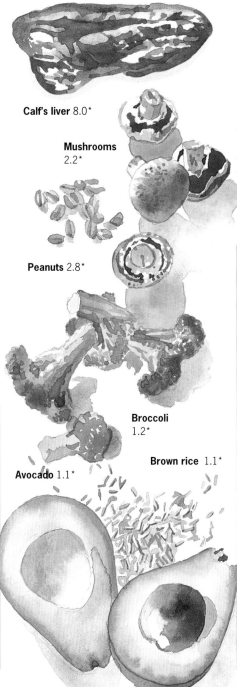

Calf's liver 8.0*

Mushrooms 2.2*

Peanuts 2.8*

Broccoli 1.2*

Brown rice 1.1*

Avocado 1.1*

SOURCES AND REQUIREMENTS

Sources
Pantothenic acid is widely distributed. Its name originates from the Greek pantothen, which roughly means "everywhere." Particularly high levels are found in liver, oily fish, whole grains, and legumes.

Dietary requirements
There is no official requirement, but 4–7 mg per day is considered adequate for the average adult.

B VITAMINS

The B group of vitamins is a collection of essential nutrients that have certain characteristics in common. All are water soluble, which means they are easily absorbed, and they are essential to the steps in the body's metabolism that lead to the release of energy from food in the diet or from body stores.

Although severe deficiencies are relatively rare, there is substantial evidence that mild or moderate deficiencies do occur and are often indicated by fatigue. People considered at risk for problems associated with shortages of B vitamins include alcoholics, the elderly, those with poor or restricted diets, and anyone suffering from chronic stress or depression or other mental disorders.

Vitamin B₆

Also known as pyridoxine, vitamin B₆ is a major player in the metabolism of amino acids and is necessary for the formation of hemoglobin in the blood, crucial for maintaining energy levels.

THE B VITAMINS AND PSYCHIATRIC PROBLEMS

Many studies have examined the possibility of vitamin B deficiencies in people with psychiatric problems. A doctor at Northwick Park Hospital in London, for example, showed that patients diagnosed with anxiety, depression, or schizophrenia had a 50 percent chance of being deficient in one or more B vitamins. He linked depression particularly with vitamin B₂ and B₆ deficiencies. Some physicians now prescribe B complex supplements for those suffering from mental illnesses.

B vitamins are also prescribed by doctors for relieving a few of the symptoms of premenstrual syndrome, including fluid retention and depression.

Vitamin B₆ is important for many different functions in the body but primarily for its roles in proper nerve function, synthesis of red blood cells, and the metabolizing of proteins, carbohydrates, and certain fats. Deficiency may adversely affect the conversion of the amino acid tryptophan into niacin, thus influencing the biochemical status and contributing to depression and other psychological imbalances.

Physical symptoms of deficiency include itchy, scaling skin, especially around the eyes, nose, and mouth; muscle weakness; weight loss; smooth, red tongue; irritability; and depressed immune function.

A number of studies have shown supplements of vitamin B₆ to be helpful in treating mild depression, particularly when associated with PMS (see box, left). It has also proved effective in relieving carpal tunnel syndrome, a painful compression of the nerve that runs between the ligaments and bones of the wrist. Another useful application of pyri-

SOURCES AND REQUIREMENTS

Sources
Vitamin B₆ is found widely in many foods but particularly in meat, fish, poultry, eggs, soybeans, green leafy vegetables, potatoes, and whole grains.

Dietary requirements
The RDAs in the U.S. are 2 mg for males, 1.6 mg for females. Canada has no RNI.

doxine supplements is in prevention of nerve dysfunction in diabetes.

Supplementation has to be carefully controlled, however, because in high doses, especially over a long period of time, this vitamin can be toxic. Symptoms of excess include drowsiness, tingling sensations or loss of feeling in the fingers and toes, loss of muscle coordination, and damage to nerve cells.

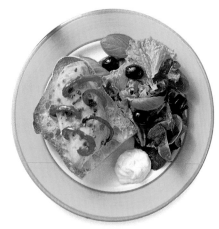

GRILLED CHICKEN AND PEPPER ROSETTI *Marinate skinless, boneless chicken breast in lemon juice, garlic, and olive oil for a few hours. Place under a hot broiler with slices of bell pepper until cooked. Serve on toast accompanied by salad greens, basil, olives, and a dollop of mayonnaise. Poultry, leafy greens, and bread are good sources of vitamin B₆.*

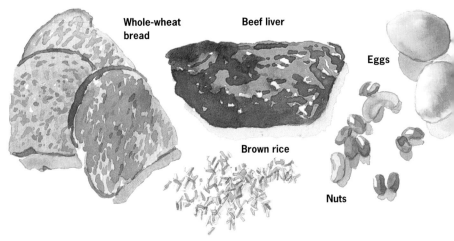

Whole-wheat bread • Beef liver • Eggs • Brown rice • Nuts

Vitamin B₁₂

Vitamin B₁₂, sometimes referred to as cobalamin, is found primarily in animal foods. It is essential to humans for the production of red blood cells, DNA, RNA, and myelin, a protective sheath for nerve fibers.

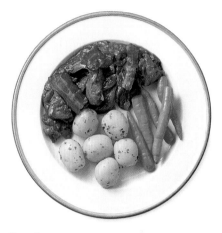

Vitamin B₁₂ in the diet is absorbed in the lower part of the small intestine, but it requires the presence of hydrochloric acid and a compound known as intrinsic factor, both produced by the stomach, and the pancreatic enzyme trypsin, produced by the small intestine.

Conditions affecting the stomach and the lower part of the small intestine can cause a vitamin B₁₂ deficiency. However, because this vitamin is stored in the liver and kidneys and the body's stores can last for three to six years, a clinically obvious deficiency, known as pernicious anemia, takes some time to become evident.

The people most prone to vitamin B₁₂ deficiency are the elderly because hydrochloric acid and the intrinsic factor decrease with age. Persons with age-related dementia have been greatly helped by supplementation with vitamin B₁₂. Treatment is with either injections or pills. Injections are usually given daily for a week and then once a month for life.

CALF'S LIVER AND BACON
Fry strips of bacon with a sliced onion. When nearly cooked, add strips of liver and fry for 2 minutes. Make a gravy by stirring a tablespoonful of flour into the juices and then adding a little stock.

SOURCES AND REQUIREMENTS

Sources
The best sources of vitamin B₁₂ are liver and shellfish, especially clams. Other good sources are meat, fish, dairy products, and eggs. While vitamin B₁₂ does occur in some vegetable foods, such as fermented soy products and sea vegetables, it is not certain how well the vitamin from these sources is utilized, if at all, by the human body. Anyone on a vegan diet, which includes no animal foods, should consider eating products fortified with the vitamin or taking a supplement.

Dietary requirements
The requirements for vitamin B₁₂ are minimal, particularly since the body conserves most of the vitamin. For adults 2 mcg per day is the RDA in the United States. The RNI in Canada is 1 mcg per day.

*mcg per 100 g

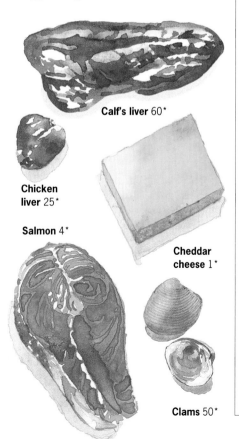

Calf's liver 60*

Chicken liver 25*

Salmon 4*

Cheddar cheese 1*

Clams 50*

SYMPTOMS OF DEFICIENCY

A long-term shortage of vitamin B₁₂ results in an anemia that has many of the same symptoms produced by a deficiency of folic acid or iron, typically, exhaustion, shortness of breath on exertion, and pale skin. There are also characteristic changes in the nervous system, including numbness and tingling in the hands and feet, clumsiness, and difficulty in walking. A blood test will reveal large, immature red blood cells (which is also true of folic acid anemia).

Because vegans are prone to B₁₂ deficiency, they may be advised to have their blood tested periodically for levels of vitamin B₁₂ (not just large red blood cells). Early treatment for deficiency is vital to prevent serious and potentially permanent damage to the nervous system.

▼▼

Folic acid

Folic acid, also known as folate and folacin, is vital for proper functioning of the central nervous system; production of red blood cells, DNA, and RNA; and the synthesis of certain amino acids.

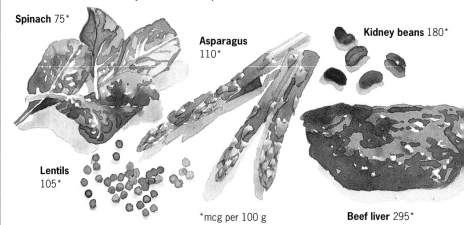

Spinach 75*
Asparagus 110*
Kidney beans 180*
Lentils 105*
*mcg per 100 g
Beef liver 295*

FOLIC ACID AND PREGNANCY

Folic acid is particularly important before and during pregnancy. This is because of its role in cell division and DNA synthesis. With insufficient folic acid, cells do not divide properly, and fetal development may be impaired. This can lead to birth defects, including spina bifida, in which the spine doesn't develop properly, and anacephaly, a malformed brain. Pregnant women are therefore advised to take supplements to avoid deficiency. (There is no evidence to suggest that taking more folic acid than needed improves fetal development.) Premature infants are also given folic acid supplements to ensure stable and healthy growth.

Folic acid, vital to many metabolic processes, is absorbed from food and transported to the liver, where it is metabolized and stored. The metabolism of folic acid and vitamin B_{12} are closely linked.

Oral contraceptives interfere with absorption of folacin. So also does alcohol, and alcoholics are very prone to a deficiency of this vitamin. Cooking usually destroys about half of it in vegetables.

Mild folic acid deficiency is fairly common in populations worldwide; symptoms include insomnia, irritability, and recurrent mouth ulcers. Severe folic acid deficiencies show up as anemia, characterized by tiredness, shortness of breath, and pale skin, as well as depression and, in extreme cases, nerve damage. Cracking at the corners of the mouth has been linked with folic acid deficiency, but this is also a sign of deficiencies in vitamins B_2, B_6, and iron. The main groups at risk of deficiency are pregnant and breast-feeding women and infants.

SOURCES AND REQUIREMENTS

Sources
The best sources include liver, nuts, whole-grain cereals, avocados, and leafy green vegetables (the name folic comes from the word foliage). Bread and some other foods are also fortified with it.

Dietary requirements
The USRDA is 200 mcg per day for men and 180 mcg for women. The Canadian RNI is 220–230 mcg for men, 180–200 mcg for women. Women who are planning a pregnancy should take a supplement of 400 mcg every day and continue until they are in their 12th week.

Folic acid antagonists, such as methotrexate, are used in chemotherapy to prevent the folic acid from synthesizing cancer cells, thus slowing spread of the disease. This may also cause deficiency symptoms.

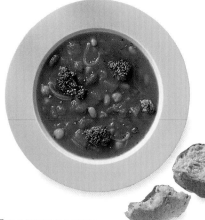

TUSCAN BEAN SOUP
Chop and lightly sauté some broccoli, onion, and garlic in a large saucepan. Add a can of chopped tomatoes and some cooked beans, boiling water, chopped herbs, and a splash of red wine. Season and simmer for 20 minutes. Both broccoli and beans are rich in folic acid.

▲▲

Choline

Choline, related to the B vitamins, is crucial to the metabolism of fats and the moving of cholesterol through the system. It is also an essential component of cell membranes and nerve tissue.

Choline is a constituent of lecithin, a fat emulsifier that is necessary for the proper metabolism of fats. Without choline, fats become trapped in the liver and can block metabolism, which can lead to major disorders in the liver and kidneys and massive energy loss. Choline also acts as a neurotransmitter in the brain. Low levels have been linked to poor memory and Alzheimer's disease.

Choline supplements, given in tandem with lecithin, have been shown to favorably affect brain function in people with memory loss or certain neurological or mood disorders.

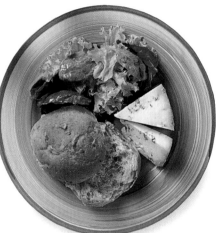

MIXED GREEN SALAD WITH CHEESE AND WHOLE-GRAIN ROLL
Toss a mixture of lettuce leaves and baby spinach with French dressing and serve with a wedge of your favorite cheese and a whole-grain roll. All of these ingredients provide choline.

SOURCES AND REQUIREMENTS

Sources
Choline is abundant in a range of foods, particularly eggs, fish, meat, legumes, and dairy products but also whole-grain cereals and some vegetables. From foods that contain complete protein, the body can also make sufficient choline to meet its normal needs, so defficiency of this nutrient is rare.

Dietary requirements
There are no recommended daily allowances. However, supplemental megadoses can be dangerous, leading to gastric, cardiovascular, and nerve problems. Supplements also produce an unpleasant fishy odor on the breath.

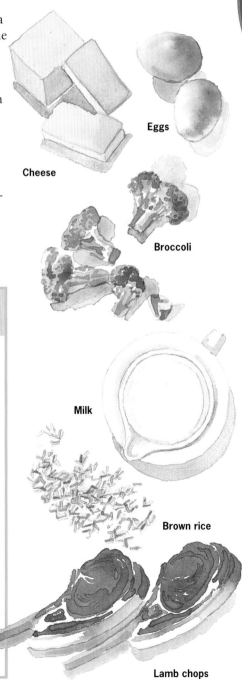

Cheese

Eggs

Broccoli

Milk

Brown rice

Lamb chops

THE MOOD-ALTERING INDUSTRY

There is a growing interest in the food and beverage industries to develop products with psychoactive effects. Choline is thought to have the potential, when channeled properly, to change a person's mood because of its ability to raise levels of neurotransmitters and thus encourage feelings of contentment and relaxation.

A company in the United States has advertised soft drinks that "allow you to take control of your neurochemistry," including one called Gourmet Choline Cooler. It cannot be assumed, however, that the inclusion of a neurotransmitter precursor in a food or drink will endow the product with mood-altering properties.

Vitamin C

Many studies have shown a strong relationship between fatigue and intake of vitamin C. A deficiency can cause not only loss of energy but also dull, aching muscular pain in the legs.

SCURVY AND VITAMIN C DEFICIENCY

The earliest documented recognition that a nutritional deficiency of some sort could cause a lack of energy came in 1753 from Dr. James Lind, a British naval surgeon who was working with cases of scurvy in sailors. Lind observed that the first symptom was a "listlessness to action or an aversion to any sort of exercise ... much fatigue ... breathlessness and panting." He also noted that sailors under stress developed scurvy faster than those who were not, despite their similar diets. It is now well known that stress increases the body's needs for certain micronutrients, including vitamin C. Although vitamin C had not been isolated at the time, it had been observed that citrus fruits prevented scurvy, and they were therefore regularly issued to sailors.

Vitamin C, also known as ascorbic acid, has many roles in the body. It is required for making and maintaining collagen, the connective tissue that holds body cells together. It also promotes healing of wounds and burns, builds strong teeth and bones, strengthens blood vessels, and helps maintain the immune system. Vitamin C has an effect on energy because it is involved in the production of a substance called carnitine (see opposite page).

Vitamin C is easily destroyed by cooking, and people living in institutions, including nursing homes, are at risk of deficiency because of overcooked vegetables and insufficient fresh fruit. As little as 5 mg per day will prevent scurvy, a disease characterized by sores, loose teeth, and spongy, bleeding gums, but mild deficiency can occur easily and may cause depression, lethargy, easy bruising, aches and pains, particularly in the legs, and impaired immune function.

SOURCES AND REQUIREMENTS

Sources
Among fruits, kiwis and papayas are the best sources of vitamin C, followed by citrus fruits, berries, and cantaloupe. Peppers, cauliflower, and broccoli are good vegetable sources.

Dietary requirements
In the U.S. the RDA is 60 mg for all adults; in Canada, 40 mg for men, 30 mg for women. Some experts believe that more would be optimal.

People who smoke or drink a lot of alcohol are believed to break down vitamin C more quickly and therefore need more than the daily requirement. Additional amounts are needed also during periods of chronic stress or acute illness or infection and for tissue repair after an operation or serious burn.

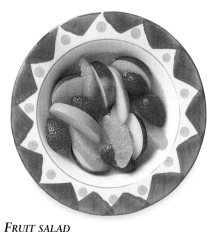

FRUIT SALAD
Mix six halved strawberries with an apple and an orange cut into bite-sized pieces. Add fruit juice and honey to taste. Strawberries are an excellent source of vitamin C; oranges are also rich in this nutrient; apples contain a modest amount.

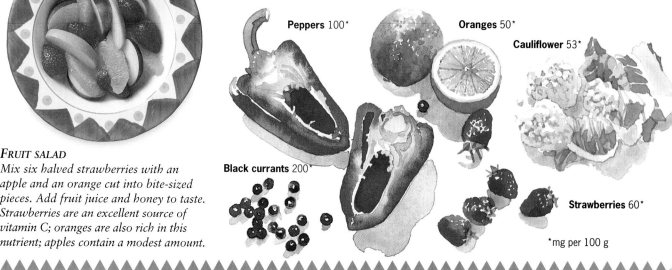

Peppers 100*

Oranges 50*

Cauliflower 53*

Black currants 200*

Strawberries 60*

*mg per 100 g

Carnitine

Carnitine is an amino acid that plays an important role in energy production, enabling the muscle cells to convert fat into energy. When carnitine levels are low, there will be a reduction in muscle function.

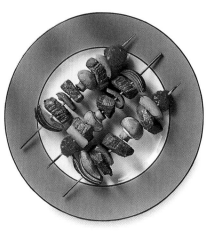

Carnitine enables fatty acids in the body to cross into the inner membrane of mitochondria (tiny energy factories within each cell) so they can be transformed into energy. The more carnitine there is in the system, the more efficiently fat is turned into energy.

Carnitine synthesis requires adequate vitamin C and iron, and people with a poor diet or a high alcohol intake may suffer from a deficiency of either of these, leading to poor carnitine synthesis. Formula-fed babies may also lack carnitine, so formulas are often fortified with it.

Carnitine deficiency has been linked to heart problems because the heart tissues prefer to utilize the fatty acids transferred by carnitine rather than other amino acids. Heart conditions have been improved with a high-carnitine diet or supplements.

GRILLED KEBABS
Cut thick lean beefsteak or lamb into cubes; skewer them along with pieces of bell pepper, onion, mushrooms, and tomatoes. Grill or broil for 15 minutes, turning occasionally. Beef is a rich source of carnitine.

Green beans

Ham

Cheddar cheese

Lamb chops

Eggs

Milk

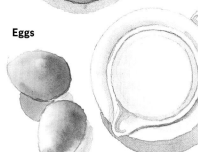

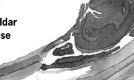

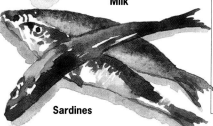

Sardines

SOURCES AND REQUIREMENTS

Sources
Carnitine is found largely in animal foods, chiefly in beef and lamb—the redder the meat, the higher the carnitine content. It is also available in dairy products and fish. The body can make its own carnitine from two amino acids found in fish, dairy products, and legumes.

Dietary requirements
Precisely how much carnitine people require is not yet known. The body produces a certain amount, and on average, most people obtain 50–100 mg a day from food.

CARNITINE AND ATHLETIC PERFORMANCE

Several scientific research programs have shown that supplements of L-carnitine can help athletes optimize their performance legally. Carnitine improves athletic performance by increasing the body's oxygen uptake and fitness rating. It can also reduce the tendency of the body to create lactic acid (a buildup of lactic acid results in tiredness and muscle cramps).

Iron

Iron is an essential part of the proteins hemoglobin and myoglobin, which transport oxygen in the red blood cells and store it in muscles. It is also a vital component of many of the body's enzyme systems.

Watercress
1.6*

Eggs 2.0*

Dried apricots
4.1*

Plain chocolate
2.4*

Calf's liver
14*

*mg per 100 g

FACTORS THAT INHIBIT IRON ABSORPTION

Tea and coffee taken with meals can inhibit the amount of iron that is absorbed. It is best to wait for at least 1½ hours after an iron-rich meal before drinking these beverages.

Calcium impairs iron absorption because it competes for the same receptor sites in the body. People who use calcium supplements or antacids should not take them with iron-rich meals.

The phytate, or phytic acid, content of food also hinders iron absorption. Found in nuts, legumes, and bran, phytate binds not only with iron but also with phosporous, zinc, and calcium during digestion and reduces the amount absorbed. Insufficient hydrochloric acid in the stomach, common in the elderly, is another inhibitor of iron absorption.

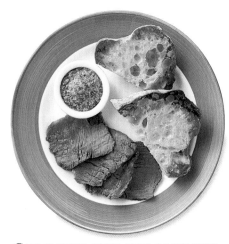

GARLIC BREAD WITH COLD ROAST BEEF Lightly toast slices of Italian bread. Rub each slice with garlic and brush with olive oil. Return to the broiler for a minute and serve hot with thinly sliced, cold roast beef, which is rich in iron.

The diets in developed countries generally include adequate iron. Still, deficiencies do occur, usually as a result of chronic blood loss or poor ability to absorb iron. Pregnant women and those with heavy periods, strict vegetarians, and people who have a poor diet are particularly at risk for deficiency. Symptoms of iron-deficiency anemia include tiredness, sore tongue, cracks at the corners of the mouth, and palpitations. Children with anemia can suffer from learning difficulties and may have impaired physical development.

The absorption of iron from food is affected by many dietary factors (see box, left). Heme iron, the form found in meat, poultry, fish, and eggs, is more available to the body; 20 to 30 percent is absorbed. Iron from plant foods, called nonheme, is poorly absorbed, and only 5 to 15 percent is available. Consuming nonheme iron with vitamin C or a little meat increases its absorption.

Chronic fatigue, a typical sign of iron deficiency, can also signal iron overload, a serious condition that can cause irreversible heart and liver damage. Other symptoms of iron overload include joint and intestinal pain, jaundice, and an irregular heartbeat. Many people also develop abnormally ruddy skin. Iron overload is most often caused by an inherited metabolic disorder but can result as well from taking potent supplements without the supervision of a doctor, dietitian, or nutritionist.

SOURCES AND REQUIREMENTS

Sources
Rich sources of heme iron are liver, red meat, seafood, and poultry. Foods high in nonheme iron include legumes and dark leafy greens.

Dietary requirements
Men and postmenopausal women need 9–10 mg daily, a menstruating woman 13–15 mg, and a pregnant woman 20–30 mg.

Tryptophan

Tryptophan is an essential amino acid needed daily for growth and repair. It is also known to be a mood enhancer and is important for the relief of stress, anxiety, and depression.

Tryptophan is converted in the brain to niacin (vitamin B_3) and serotonin, a neurotransmitter that induces sleepiness and a feeling of calmness, promoting relaxation and alleviation of stress. However, getting high levels of tryptophan into the brain is not as easy as simply eating plenty of tryptophan-rich foods. Foods that contain complete protein, such as milk, poultry, red meat, and eggs, are high in tryptophan but also in other amino acids that compete for the same entry point to the brain. A high-protein diet can actually reduce the amount of serotonin produced by the brain. On the other hand, after a meal high in complex carbohydrates, more tryptophan reaches the brain and is converted to serotonin.

Tryptophan has been studied for use in the treatment of depression and PMS, although its effectiveness has not always been consistent. Its benefits are enhanced when it is combined with vitamins B_3 and B_6.

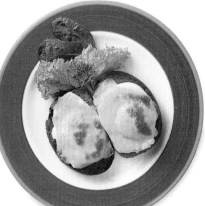

EGGS BENEDICT
Poach two eggs and lightly toast some bread. Make a hollandaise sauce by gently heating and stirring an egg yolk, 2 teaspoons water, and 1 teaspoon lemon juice until the mixture thickens slightly. Add 25 g (2 tbsp) butter, stirring it in a little at a time. When creamy, pour the sauce over the poached eggs and brown quickly under a hot broiler.

*mg per 100 g

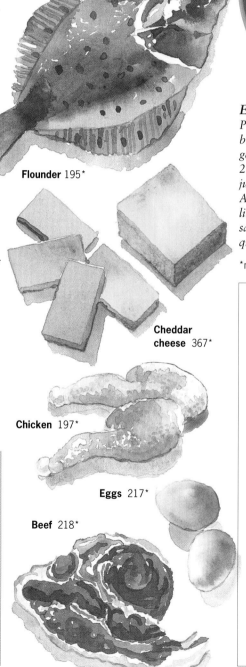

Flounder 195*

Cheddar cheese 367*

Chicken 197*

Eggs 217*

Beef 218*

SOURCES AND REQUIREMENTS

Sources
Tryptophan is available in foods that contain complete protein, such as meat, poultry, fish, eggs, and milk.

Dietary requirements
There are no daily recommendations. The sale of supplements is not approved in the United States.

TYROSINE

Tyrosine is an amino acid that, like tryptophan, may enhance mood. It is essential for the synthesis of adrenaline, nor-adrenaline, thyroid hormones, and the brown skin pigment melanin. Found in all food proteins, it becomes raised in the blood plasma in relation to other amino acids after a high-protein meal. It has been suggested that this might affect the production of neurotrans-mitters like noradrenaline and dopamine. Research has shown that some depressed people have low levels of tyrosine and, when given tyrosine supplements, their neurotransmitter production is apparently enhanced and mood improves.

Zinc

Zinc is recognized as a very important nutrient for energy balance. It is involved either directly or indirectly in a wide range of metabolic processes that affect energy levels.

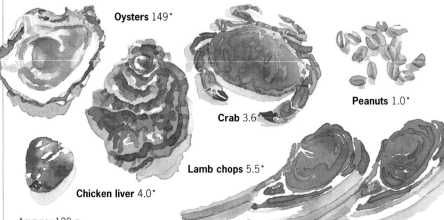

Oysters 149*

Crab 3.6*

Peanuts 1.0*

Lamb chops 5.5*

Chicken liver 4.0*

*mg per 100 g

ZINC AND THE IMMUNE SYSTEM

Many studies have shown zinc to be important in maintaining the immune system. In 1992 a Canadian research team gave zinc to a group of elderly people. Those who received the supplement experienced only half the number of days troubled by acute infections and required half the amount of antibiotics compared to those who did not take zinc. Also, some in the zinc group had evidence of mild nutritional deficiencies that cleared up.

Another study showed that taking a zinc supplement regularly during the period of a cold, starting within 24 hours of the first symptoms, significantly reduced (by almost half) the duration of symptoms.

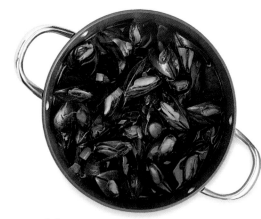

MUSSELS SAILOR STYLE
Sauté a chopped onion, a chopped celery stalk, and a few crushed cloves of garlic in a tablespoon of olive oil. Add 1 kg (2¼ lb) of scrubbed mussels in their shells, 240 ml (2 cups) of boiling water, chopped parsley, and 4 tbsp white wine. Bring to a boil, cover, and simmer for 10 minutes. Serve with French bread. Seafood is a good source of zinc.

Zinc is essential to a great many of the body's functions, including the metabolism of proteins, carbohydrates, and fats. It is needed for normal growth and sexual function and to make DNA and RNA. It is a component of some 70 enzymes; aids in the healing of wounds; and plays a major role in the proper functioning of the immune system.

Zinc deficiency increases susceptibility to infection. It can also lead to slow growth, infertility, hair loss, skin problems, impaired nerves, diarrhea, and poor wound healing. Studies have shown that a lack of zinc affects muscle strength and endurance as well; vigorous exercise seems to increase the body's requirement for the mineral.

Zinc supplements have benefited sufferers of arthritis, acne, prostate problems, and infertility. However, they should never be taken without a doctor's guidance. Excessive zinc—first signaled by nausea, vomiting, and muscle pain—can cause kidney failure, atherosclerosis, and damage

---

SOURCES AND REQUIREMENTS

Sources
By far the best dietary sources are oysters and other seafood. Red meat, nuts, seeds, eggs, yogurt, and whole-grain and fortified cereals are also high in zinc.

Dietary requirements
The RDA is 15 mg for men, 12 mg for women. In Canada the RNI is 12 mg for men, 9 mg for women.

---

to the heart. Zinc lozenges, used for a short period to ease a sore throat and reduce the severity and duration of cold symptoms, are generally safe. They are most effective when taken at the first sign of illness.

The amount of phytate in the diet affects absorption of zinc (see box, page 106). Citric acid and the sweeteners sorbitol and mannitol reduce the effectiveness of zinc lozenges.

Coenzyme Q10

Coenzyme Q10 is a critical component in the breakdown of fat into energy and production of energy within cells. It was first identified in the late 1950s in the United States.

Coenzyme Q10 (coQ10) is also known as ubiquinone (derived from the word *ubiquitous*) because it is found in almost all living cells. It can be obtained from food or synthesized in the body from two amino acids plus the B vitamins and vitamin C. Dietary sources include most animal and plant foods.

CoQ10 can be regarded as the spark plug that ignites the fuel in the mitochondria and so produces energy. A deficiency of the coenzyme results in a reduction in energy and a slowing of metabolic processes.

Levels of coQ10 decrease with age and certain diseases, and supplements have improved the conditions (see box, right). There is some evidence that coQ10 may be useful also in helping people to lose weight.

*mg per 100 g

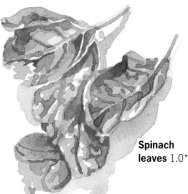

Spinach leaves 1.0*

Soy oil 9.2*

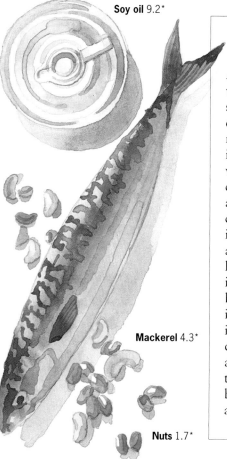

Mackerel 4.3*

Nuts 1.7*

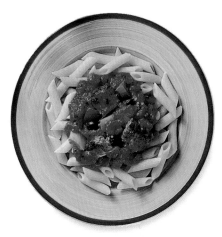

SARDINE AND OLIVE PASTA
Sauté a chopped onion and bell pepper until soft and add a 784 g (28 oz) can of chopped tomatoes, a can of sardines, and some minced herbs and halved black olives. Heat and blend the mixture thoroughly, breaking up the sardines. Serve over 450 g (1 lb) of cooked pasta.

SOURCES AND REQUIREMENTS

Sources
Almost everything we eat contains various forms of coQ10. Especially good sources include soy products, nuts, seeds, leafy green vegetables, meat, poultry, and oily fish, such as tuna, trout, and sardines.

Recommended intake
A recommended daily allowance has not been determined. Supplements given for treating certain diseases usually range between 50 and 150 mg per day but should be taken only with a doctor's advice.

COENZYME Q10 AND AGING

As we grow older, our ability to ward off infection and diseases such as cancer and arthritis decreases. This decline is related to the strength of the immune system. Experiments with mice revealed that coenzyme Q10 decreases with age. With supplementation of coQ10, the life span of the mice increased, probably because of a healthier immune system. A large amount of evidence indicates that coQ10 has a beneficial effect on a number of illnesses associated with aging in humans, including heart disease, high blood pressure, and periodontal disease. Body tissue levels of coQ10 depend both on dietary intake and the amount made within the body.

Magnesium

Magnesium helps to maintain the electrical balance of the body's tissues and is thought to be of particular importance in preventing energy problems. Some cases of fatigue can be alleviated by a high-magnesium diet.

MAGNESIUM AS A CURE FOR FATIGUE

The link between magnesium and fatigue was first discovered in the 1970s, when a group of doctors in France began to prescribe magnesium supplements to people suffering from spasmophilia, which has symptoms similar to those of magnesium deficiency—aching, twitching muscles, headaches, and mental disturbances. A team of doctors in Southampton, England, found in the 1980s that giving magnesium supplements to chronic fatigue patients whose magnesium levels were below normal brought an improvement in 80 percent of cases. Further research has not substantiated a conclusive link between energy levels and magnesium, but it is often used to help relieve chronic fatigue when deficiency seems to be a factor.

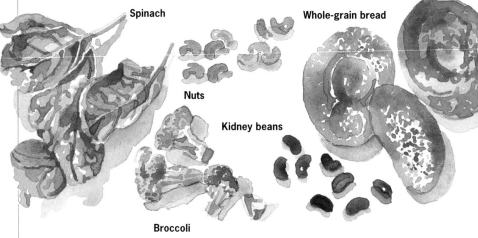

Spinach

Whole-grain bread

Nuts

Kidney beans

Broccoli

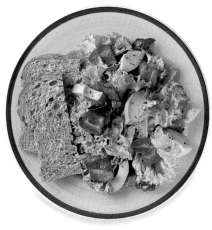

WARM BACON AND AVOCADO SALAD
Dice and fry two strips of bacon until crisp. Scatter the bacon over a salad made with mixed greens, avocado, and tomato. Serve with whole-wheat bread.

Magnesium is vital for strong bones and teeth and the effective action of many enzymes; a lack can disrupt the operation of the body's nerves and muscles and lead to poor functioning of the major organs, particularly the heart. Because magnesium is stored in the body in large quantities, however, deficiencies are rare. When they do occur, most cases are the result of digestive disorders, illness, severe weight loss, alcoholism, or persistent diarrhea and vomiting. Certain drugs, such as diuretics, can cause a deficiency and are a leading cause of magnesium-related troubles in elderly people.

Because so many bodily functions rely on magnesium, a deficiency may show itself in a variety of ways. A reduction in muscle efficiency is common, often associated with muscle fatigue, twitches, and spasms. Nausea and vomiting, personality changes, apathy, heart arrhythmia, and nerve disorders may also occur.

Supplements can raise magnesium levels and boost energy in patients

SOURCES AND REQUIREMENTS

Sources
Magnesium is plentiful in many foods, including legumes, leafy green vegetables, nuts, seeds, avocados, and whole-grain products.

Dietary requirements
The RDA (U.S.) is 350 mg for adult men, 280 mg for women. The RNI (Canada) is 230–250 mg for men, 200–210 mg for women.

who were previously deficient. They are also beneficial for controlling some cases of high blood pressure and in the prevention and treatment of osteoporosis. However, magnesium supplements can be dangerous in high doses; treatment should be monitored by a doctor. Diarrhea, nausea, and vomiting are signs of magnesium excess; continued overdosing can lead to paralysis.

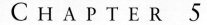

CHAPTER 5

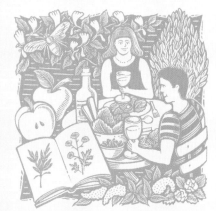

A VITAL MIND AND BODY

*Energizing both your mind and
body is key to improving your overall
health and well-being. Through regular physical
exercise you can increase the efficiency of your body
in producing energy and boost your mobility and
vitality. On a different level, practicing relaxation
and stress reduction techniques can improve
your mental energy and your ability to
cope with life's ups and downs.*

REGULAR EXERCISE FOR ENERGY

Regular exercise can bring dramatic improvements to energy levels, improving blood flow, body functioning, and oxygen supply and revitalizing mental attitude.

The more active a person is, the more energy he or she will have for living. The body and mind need energy for repair and rejuvenation and to deal with the stresses and strains of normal activities. A healthy body will have sufficient energy not only to keep itself in good repair but also to cope with the additional energy demands of work and recreation. As soon as energy levels drop, the body is less able to look after itself and to create more energy, which leads eventually to a downward spiral of fatigue and poor health. Regular exercise can help prevent you from falling into this kind of negative spiral.

OXYGEN AND ENERGY

Breathing in oxygen is essential to human existence—so much so that our bodies give us dramatic warning signs when supplies are inadequate. For example, if you exercise so strenuously that your body does not have enough oxygen to meet its needs, you may experience severe muscle cramps that prevent you from continuing the exercise. Similarly, if your brain is inadequately supplied with oxygen, you may feel confused and dizzy and even lose consciousness. The dependability of your oxygen supply is linked to the efficiency of your cardiovascular system, and regular aerobic exercise is the only way to strengthen the heart, lungs, and circulation.

Aerobic exercise includes any physical activity that demands the transportation of large amounts of oxygen by the blood to the working muscles for sustained periods. Running, cycling, swimming, aerobic dancing, and brisk walking all require such sustained muscle activity. If

FULL DRIVE AHEAD
Doing exercise can be an ideal way to focus on a different aspect of your abilities and refresh yourself to face everyday challenges.

continued for at least 12 minutes at a time, they will raise your pulse rate and provide an effective aerobic workout. By contrast, activities such as weightlifting or sprinting require a short burst of energy and utilize existing supplies of blood sugar in the body without the use of oxygen. This is known as anaerobic respiration, and it can be sustained for only a limited time before the muscles stop functioning.

Both aerobic and anaerobic exercise have health benefits, but it is the aerobic form that improves the body's cardiovascular functioning. Regular aerobic exercise of at least 20 minutes three times a week is advised for boosting your body's ability to create and access energy when you need it.

Oxygen and the brain

During an exercise session the body will experience increased blood flow, promoting the transporting of oxygen, the elimination of toxins, and the reduction of stress, all of which promote a rise in available energy. The increased blood flow improves the supply of oxygen to the brain, which aids healthy brain functioning. Laboratory research tests have shown that even though the brain makes up only 2 percent of the body's total weight, it utilizes 20 percent of its available oxygen. Some headaches, as well as fatigue and loss of concentration, can be the result of insufficient oxygenated blood reaching the brain.

MORE ACTIVE, MORE ENERGIZED

Interestingly, vigorous physical or mental exercise can actually make you feel more energetic rather than fatigued. This is because during physical exertion, hormones known as endorphins are released into the blood from the brain. These act as pain-killers, reduce stress, and induce a feeling of well-being. They are released so that the body or mind can continue to exert itself. If you exercise for a long period of time, for instance, in a marathon, your body produces endorphins to counteract the pain and fatigue in the muscles.

Even moderate exercise can raise the level of endorphins, thus improving your mental outlook and reducing stress, one of the most significant energy drainers. The exercise-stress link has been confirmed by a number

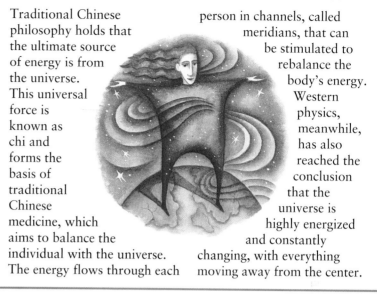

COSMIC ENERGY FORCES: *The Universe*

Traditional Chinese philosophy holds that the ultimate source of energy is from the universe. This universal force is known as chi and forms the basis of traditional Chinese medicine, which aims to balance the individual with the universe. The energy flows through each person in channels, called meridians, that can be stimulated to rebalance the body's energy. Western physics, meanwhile, has also reached the conclusion that the universe is highly energized and constantly changing, with everything moving away from the center.

of studies. For example, during the 1980s Herbert de Vries at the University of Southern California conducted an experiment with stressed and fatigued patients. He gave half of the group tranquilizers and had the other half perform some type of exercise

continued on page 116

BREATHING EXERCISE

Emotions are intricately linked to breathing, probably because of neuro-chemical reactions between the body and mind. When you cry, your physical reaction is to catch your breath and breathe rapidly and deeply. An angry person breathes quickly, building up aggression and fueling the body for physical action. You can help to relieve tension by breathing deeply and calmly.

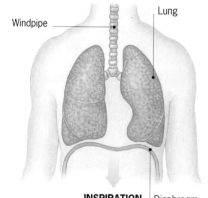

INSPIRATION | Diaphragm

1 *When you take a deep breath, or inhale, your diaphragm moves down and your chest moves outward as your lungs fill with air. Hold your breath for a few moments and feel the expansion of your lungs.*

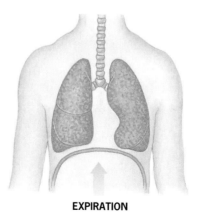

EXPIRATION

2 *Expiring involves the upward movement of the diaphragm while the chest moves inward. Practice breathing deeply for a few minutes, holding yourself upright for better air movement.*

EXERCISE FOR A BETTER BODY

Physical exercise helps energize your body in a number of ways. It can

▶ *Improve the functioning of organs, especially the heart and lungs.*

▶ *Improve blood circulation.*

▶ *Increase the energy content of every cell in the body.*

▶ *Help to cleanse the body through improving the functioning of the lymphatic system.*

▶ *Reduce physical and emotional stress.*

▶ *Reduce excess adrenaline.*

A Home Workout

Every morning when you get out of bed, put aside 5 to 10 minutes to warm up your body and get the blood flowing properly. It will not only wake you up but help you feel alert and full of energy for the rest of the day.

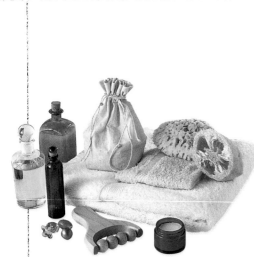

STRETCHING OUT IN THE BATH
After your home workout, take a warm bath to soothe muscles and enhance the relaxing qualities of exercise.

These stretching exercises can be performed on your own at home at any time of day. They will take from 5 to 20 minutes, depending on how long you want to spend on each routine. You may want to add your own exercises or adapt these to your particular level of fitness and flexi-

bility. There is no need to hurry, although you should make sure that your heartbeat is raised sufficiently to pump the blood around your body at a faster speed than when resting. This will improve your body's ability to transfer oxygen and food to the cells and convert them into energy.

1 *From a standing position, take a giant step forward, keeping your hands on your hips for support. Lean into the step and hold for a few seconds. Return to the standing position, then step forward with the other leg. Repeat 8 times on each side.*

2 *Lie on your back with your knees bent and feet flat on the floor. Put your right hand behind your head and reach out with your left hand to touch your right knee. Relax back to lying position. Repeat 8 times on each side.*

Hold the position for a few seconds before relaxing.

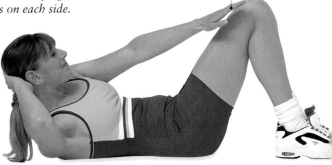

Back should be straight and upright.

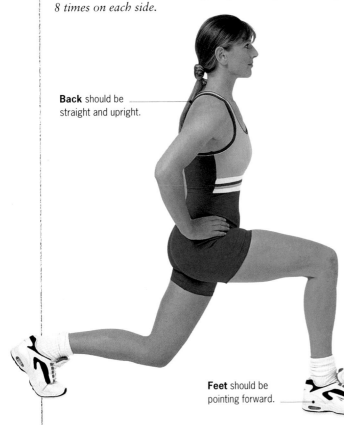

Feet should be pointing forward.

3 *Still lying on your back, put both hands behind your head and lift your legs so that your thighs are at right angles to your body and your calves are parallel to the floor. Now raise your head, neck, and shoulders off the ground, hold for a few seconds, and then relax back to the floor. Repeat 8 times.*

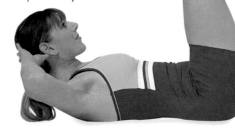

Keep your calves at a right angle to your thighs.

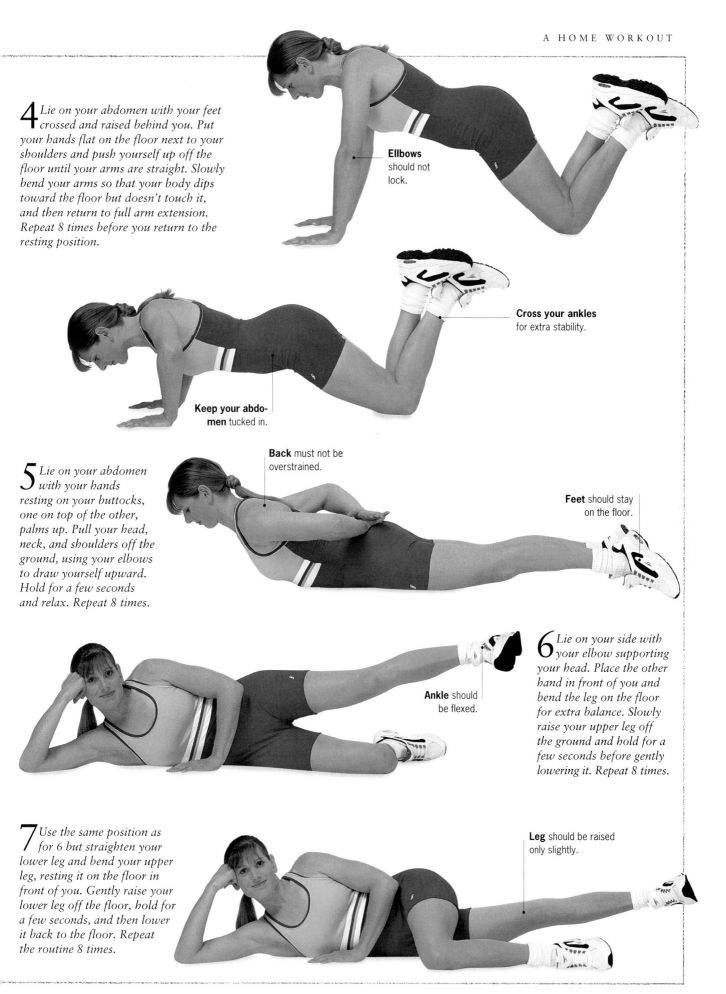

4 *Lie on your abdomen with your feet crossed and raised behind you. Put your hands flat on the floor next to your shoulders and push yourself up off the floor until your arms are straight. Slowly bend your arms so that your body dips toward the floor but doesn't touch it, and then return to full arm extension. Repeat 8 times before you return to the resting position.*

Ellbows
should not
lock.

Cross your ankles
for extra stability.

**Keep your abdo-
men** tucked in.

Back must not be
overstrained.

5 *Lie on your abdomen with your hands resting on your buttocks, one on top of the other, palms up. Pull your head, neck, and shoulders off the ground, using your elbows to draw yourself upward. Hold for a few seconds and relax. Repeat 8 times.*

Feet should stay
on the floor.

Ankle should
be flexed.

6 *Lie on your side with your elbow supporting your head. Place the other hand in front of you and bend the leg on the floor for extra balance. Slowly raise your upper leg off the ground and hold for a few seconds before gently lowering it. Repeat 8 times.*

7 *Use the same position as for 6 but straighten your lower leg and bend your upper leg, resting it on the floor in front of you. Gently raise your lower leg off the floor, hold for a few seconds, and then lower it back to the floor. Repeat the routine 8 times.*

Leg should be raised
only slightly.

every day. From the results he discovered that just a 15-minute walk every day is more relaxing and efficient in dealing with stress than any course of tranquilizers.

STRETCHING

As with all forms of exercise, stretching is an important warmup, allowing your body to adjust to the strain of physical exercise. However, stretching also provides its own energy benefits. It can help you realign your skeletal structure, release tension from your muscles, and relax your joints, leaving you ready for action and exertion. In addition, it makes you feel good, liberating you from the confines of your normal movement and allowing you to release pressures and anxieties that have been holding you back.

GETTING INTO EXERCISE

Although the health benefits of regular exercise are irrefutable, it can still be difficult to change a sedentary lifestyle to a more active

DID YOU KNOW?

An important element of Chinese Taoist philosophy is to "embrace the uncarved block of wood," meaning that you must see yourself as a new entity that has the potential to be carved into any number of forms. Do not try to fit into a rigid mold, restricting yourself with endless rules and regulations, or be led totally by others. Let your natural energy flow freely and tell you which path is best for you.

one. It may be especially hard for anyone who is suffering from fatigue. Some people find that a change is more easily achieved by fairly dramatic means, such as signing up for a year's membership at a gym. Others find it easier to make a gentle adaptation from their current lifestyle. If you remember that any form of physical activity is helpful, you should be able to integrate

ASHTANGA VINYASA YOGA

Yoga means "union," and it is the union of mind, body, and spirit that yoga aims to achieve. Regular practice of yoga will result in improved flexibility, strength, posture, and breathing and increased energy, tranquility, and motivation.

Ashtanga Vinyasa yoga is a method that has been in existence for some 1,500 years. It was rediscovered in 1930 and is now practiced worldwide. Ashtanga Vinyasa yoga aims to unite physical (*hatha*) and mental (*raja*) yoga through a variety of postures, breathing, and concentration. Each posture (*asana*) should ideally be held for as long as possible to enhance muscular strength and suppleness, although for beginners this may not be advised in the initial stages. The focus is first toward alignment of the body to improve physical balance. If a body is in natural alignment, this will improve posture and decrease muscular tension. Attention is then given to specific breathing patterns, or *pranayama*, designed to stimulate the energy flow, or *prana*, in the body.

SURYANAMASKAR—SALUTE TO THE SUN

An Ashtanga Vinyasa yoga session will usually start with the Suryanamaskar—a basic exercise to harness energy. Move gradually through the positions in a flowing movement. The exercise is supposed to be done several times quite quickly so that you feel warmed up by the end. Do it more slowly if you have back problems.

1 *Stand up straight and relaxed, with your legs together and your arms at rest at your sides. Keep your head straight and your eyes looking directly forward. Relax and focus on your breathing.*

Stand upright and relaxed.

Feel the stretch through your whole body.

2 *Reach your hands up together toward the sky above you. The movement should be quite fast. Bend your head back and look up.*

more activity into the things you already do. For example, simply deciding to take a walk during your lunch hour rather than sitting in the lunchroom can make a difference, expecially if you gradually increase both the frequency of your walks and your speed. Exercise at midday can also give you a much needed energy boost for getting through the afternoon and evening. Walking up stairs rather than taking an elevator or escalator can also help improve your health.

While sitting on the sofa and watching television, you can do some simple exercises to enhance your fitness and flexibility. Try a few leg lifts, head rotations, and arm stretches. Rather than thinking of how to avoid physical effort, consider how you can maximize your exercise opportunities.

EASTERN EXERCISE TRADITIONS

Eastern systems of health have long recognized that exercise is integral to energy levels. In fact, health systems such as Ayurveda

SEX FOR ENERGY AND HEALTH

Sex is an excellent energy enhancer and can also relax you thoroughly. Not only is it a highly effective form of physical exercise, using a large range of muscles, but it is also a great mood enhancer, helping you to feel good.

▶ *Sexual activity can improve your heart and lung functions.*

▶ *For women, regular sex increases estrogen levels, improving skin and hair and correcting menstrual imbalances.*

▶ *Endorphins are released by the pituitary gland, lifting mood and countering stress.*

▶ *Touch is emotionally soothing.*

▶ *Muscles become relaxed through the sexual act and physical contact.*

▶ *Boosting the immune system, regular sex has been found to counter breast cancer development.*

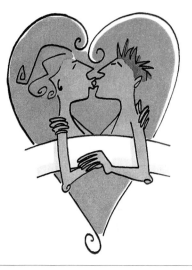

3 *Bend down from your hips, keeping your legs straight and together. Try to touch your legs with your head, although this may be difficult at first.*

Bend your knees if you cannot reach the floor.

4 *Keeping your hands on the floor (bend your knees if you cannot reach), transfer your weight onto your palms, look up, and prepare to jump or step back.*

5 *Without moving your hands, jump or step back, then gently lower your body, keeping your elbows in. Bend your arms so that your shoulders are raised just above the floor, as if to do a push-up.*

Keep your arms straight and hands flat on the floor.

6 *Roll forward onto the front of your toes and push your upper body forward and up by straightening your arms. Curl your back and look upward.*

7 *Using your hips to push up, roll back onto the soles of your feet and straighten your back, keeping your arms straight and your hands on the floor in front of you.*

Back and shoulders must be straight and stretched out.

(see page 48) and therapies like yoga, t'ai chi, and chi kung use exercise as a core feature of a complete approach to improving and balancing energy flow in the body.

Chi kung is divided into two general categories: a tranquil or meditative aspect, in which the emphasis is on concentration, visualization, and breathing; and dynamic chi kung, based on activity. Each aspect of the therapy is equally important in bringing about a proper flow of life energy in the body, often focusing on restoring energy balance (see pages 120–121). A number of experiments have indicated that chi kung benefits both the mind and the body. A research project conducted at the Shanghai Institute of Hypertension found that chi kung appeared to reduce the risk of cardiovascular disease and that this was due both to its impact on circulation and its relaxing effect. The mixture of physical exercise with uplifting meditative movements makes chi kung a remarkable therapeutic experience.

MIND–BODY LINK

The emotions and the body are intricately linked by neuropeptides, a group of chemicals that transport messages between the brain and the body. Neuropeptides are responsible for telling you when you are thirsty or hungry, for stimulating good feelings, and creating the sensation of pleasure. It has been found that breathing deeply—such as during breathing exercises or meditation—can cause a flood of emotions. This is because the part of the brain stem responsible for breathing is thickly endowed with neuropeptides and neuropeptide receptors, which cause a heightened, positive, and vital mood. Focusing on your breathing can therefore lift mood and help rebalance your energies.

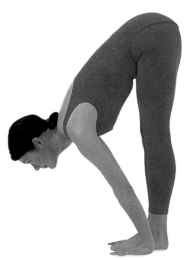

8 *Return to position 4 by jumping or walking your feet back between your hands. Straighten your back and look up.*

9 *Pull your body into your legs and adopt position 3. Once again you can bend your knees if your hands do not reach the floor.*

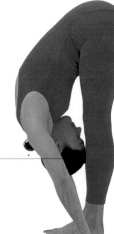

Head should ideally touch your legs.

10 *Reach your arms right up and face the sky as you did for position 2. Feel the upward stretch throughout your whole body.*

Face the sky with your hands up in the air.

Legs and feet should be together.

11 *Return to the starting position, standing straight and relaxed. Focus on your breathing and then begin the whole routine once again.*

Stand upright and relaxed.

ENERGY AND YOUR EMOTIONS

Both positive and negative emotions can sap vitality. After any intense emotional experience, the body's energy reserves are lower, and rest is needed to restore equilibrium.

When you feel an intense emotion—good or bad—your body calls upon its ability to produce "emergency hormones," which help you to cope with the need of the moment. The instant an extreme emotion is recognized, an arousal system is set off. The adrenal glands produce adrenaline, noradrenaline, and corticosteroid hormones, which begin to surge around the body, causing the muscles to tighten, the heart to beat faster, the breathing to quicken, and the blood supply for the skin to be reduced.

This action energizes the body, enabling it to respond quickly to the emotion. However, this emotional surge draws heavily upon the body's reserves, which must then be restored. Normally, the body can do this through sleep and the digestion of food, but sometimes the hormones do not know when to switch off, and you remain on a "high" far longer than necessary. This can cause insomnia and loss of appetite or a craving for sugary foods, which are stimulants that can lead to exhaustion of the adrenal glands.

continued on page 122

EMOTIONS AND YOUR ENERGY BODY CLOCK

Your nergy levels rise and fall throughout the day, depending on your emotions, stresses, and periods of rest and relaxation. When energy-building emotions are not in balance with energy-draining ones, an energy deficit results, leaving you tired and in need of rest and recuperation. Periods of intense or prolonged stress call for more relaxation than normal to rebuild the body's energy and rebalance the negative effects of stress.

A TYPICAL DAY
Every day brings a variety of emotional challenges. Making sure that you balance your emotional energies can help you to stay on top of daily stresses.

Working on a computer increases stress and energy drain.

Morning meeting creates negative stress emotions.

Going to work is unnerving: will you be late?

Morning mail brings a wedding invitation and positive emotions.

The day starts with a wake-up bath or shower to stimulate circulation.

The day ends with a light meal, helping you to unwind.

Lunch with friends gives you a chance to unwind and talk about the meeting.

Afternoon is busy being creative and getting things done, but you feel steady energy drain.

A friend calls to invite you to play squash on the weekend, giving you something to look forward to.

Relaxing at home with a yoga session eases stress and boosts your energy.

The Chi Kung Teacher

Chi kung is the cultivation of internal energy—the vital breath of life that gives us the ability to function healthily. Dance movements, some of them imitating the movements of animals and embodying their powers, are used to restore positive energy.

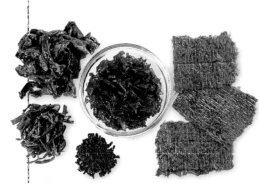

DAILY SEAWEED
Chi kung practitioners recommend eating one or two tablespoons of seaweed every day for good health. Seaweed can also be taken in tablet form.

DURING A CLASS
The moves are first demonstrated by the teacher, who then helps the class members through each aspect of the movement.

Chi kung is practiced by performing specific movements in coordination with breathing and meditation techniques. The exercises aim to energize and rebalance the body, uniting body, mind, and spirit in a natural, unrestricted way. Practicing these exercises regularly can help you find the energy to enjoy a happier, healthier, and less restricted life.

What happens during a chi kung session?
A chi kung session takes place in silence to help the mind focus completely on the exercises and the movement and restoration of energy. The teacher will lead a warm-up routine, including breathing exercises, posture adjustments, and a variety of smooth-flowing exercises that gently loosen the joints and create body heat. The chi kung exercises are then taught, mostly step by step, with the teacher clearly demonstrating the exercises and giving explanations regarding what to focus on and specific details of each movement.

Because all the movements are performed at a very slow pace, it is possible to follow the teacher through some of the movements, then he or she will watch and correct your posture afterward. You may be asked to retain a posture for several minutes, focusing your mind during this time on your breathing. Another element that may be incorporated is self-massage, which helps to stimulate the flow of chi through your body. If you are practicing with a group of people, it is usual to perform all the exercises in a circle.

What qualifications does a chi kung teacher have?
There are no official qualifications; length of practice and expertise are the most common indicators of a teacher's skill. In China a committee of masters can qualify a person who is well practiced in chi kung to become a master.

What are the benefits of chi kung?
Chi kung exercises can lead to remarkable improvements in your health, as well as make you feel livelier and happier. The aim of a chi kung session is to relax, energize, and restore balance to both your

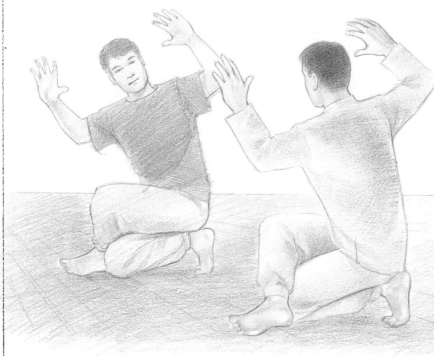

Origins

Elements of chi kung have been used for thousands of years. Ancient cave paintings in China depict dance moves that imitate the characteristics of animals; these later became the more structured energy exercises incorporated into the Taoist spiritual tradition, which encourages harmony between the individual and the natural world. The *Taoist Canon* (a treatise of 1,120 volumes) contains all the early texts of chi kung, which were subsequently influenced by Indian yoga and Tibetan Buddhism. Chi kung continues to be practiced up to the present day, although it was discouraged by the Chinese Communist regime for much of the 20th century. Dr Qian Xue-sen, a scientist educated in the United States, returned to China during the Cultural Revolution (1966–76) and reestablished the tradition.

body and your mind. To achieve these benefits, the session incorporates a variety of specific exercises, including stretching, breathing, and mental exercises, which stimulate the flow of chi. According to the principles of traditional Chinese medicine, stagnant chi in the body is the chief cause of illness. Chi kung is designed to help the chi circulate more efficiently and thus restock the body with fresh energy.

You should be able to feel the positive effects of chi kung even after the first session. One of the initial benefits is the acquiring of a sense of calmness and clarity of mind. In the long term, chi kung can improve your emotional health and stability, and it has also been known to help combat specific psychological and physical illnesses.

What are the "Three Treasures" and how are they used?

Central to the philosophy of Taoism, from which chi kung derives, is the concept of the Three Treasures. The first of these is *jing,* which is both sexual energy and the germ of life. The second is *chi,* the omnipresent energy of life. The last is *shen,* which means "stretch" and symbolizes the subtle energy of the spirit, stretching up toward the universe. These treasures have been likened to the energies of the mind, body, and spirit. Each is a crucial part of the whole, and the idea is to refine jing to chi, refine chi to shen, and ultimately refine shen and return to the void. The void is a state of empty clear-mindedness—your original mind untouched by concepts or images—and this is the ultimate goal of practicing chi kung. Chi kung uses movement to effect this transformation, aiming to help you understand each state through breathing and physical awareness and balance.

WHAT YOU CAN DO AT HOME

Stand with your feet a little more than hip width apart and legs slightly bent at the knee. Feel your spine lengthen and come into alignment. Relax the shoulders and face muscles. Start to breathe deeply. Inhale through the nose and focus on the breath going into the lower part of the stomach. Spread your arms out and imagine them as branches growing naturally into the outside world. Exhale and imagine your feet growing roots that penetrate the earth, grounding you and giving you strength. Practice for at least five minutes. This exercise is a good way to rejuvenate the body's circulation.

STANDING LIKE A TREE
This simple exercise can help to promote a sense of being rooted. It can be helpful during moments of anxiety or trauma or for promoting general relaxation.

How can chi kung help with emotional problems?

Stress and anxiety build up when your emotions are suppressed in order to cope with everyday demands. Chi kung breathing exercises draw attention to your breath, and this process clears your mind and creates an awareness that allows you to tune in to how your inner self is feeling about life and identify any problems. This is known as "listening to the energy." By freeing your deeper feelings, you will find your inner self less burdened and restored to emotional health.

Chi kung thus aims to resolve emotional issues, some of which you may not even know you have. The stress relief will unburden your muscles and body and slow your pulse and heartbeat, improving physical health and energy. The feeling of emotional calm and balance experienced with chi kung also has an invigorating effect, replenishing your energy and leaving you feeling refreshed.

Focus on your breath traveling right down to your navel.

COSMIC ENERGY FORCES: *The Sun*

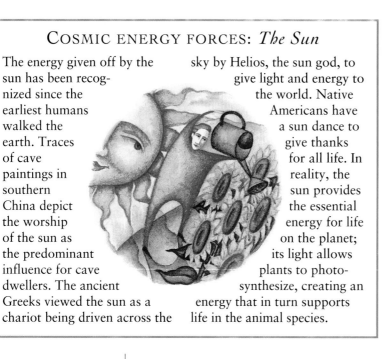

The energy given off by the sun has been recognized since the earliest humans walked the earth. Traces of cave paintings in southern China depict the worship of the sun as the predominant influence for cave dwellers. The ancient Greeks viewed the sun as a chariot being driven across the sky by Helios, the sun god, to give light and energy to the world. Native Americans have a sun dance to give thanks for all life. In reality, the sun provides the essential energy for life on the planet; its light allows plants to photosynthesize, creating an energy that in turn supports life in the animal species.

EMOTIONAL STRESSES AND ENERGY

Stress experts have categorized the three different kinds of stress—mental, physical, and emotional—into three sequential phases. Phase one harnesses the body's energy reserves; phase two utilizes these reserves; and phase three drains them further and leads to exhaustion. Emotional stress is often prolonged in phase three, and it drains the energy stores more than any other form of stress, affecting physical and mental as well as emotional reserves.

As the body struggles to cope with the demands of intense emotions, other feelings tend to get lost; a sense of humor and talent for enjoying life may disappear. Behavioral changes may also occur; for example, a once happy-go-lucky person may become quiet and withdrawn. An individual may not notice such changes in himself but others will. Motivation is also reduced and tasks become harder to perform. Concentration is impaired and planning becomes difficult. Anxiety about the inability to cope in all the different areas of life distresses the sufferer further. The end result is complete exhaustion, and when the body's energy reserves are exhausted, illnesses take hold.

The body's ability to protect itself and fight infection is governed by the immune system, which is directly controlled by the mind and the way that you are feeling emotionally. Negative emotions and thought patterns reduce the efficiency of the body's defense system because they drain energy that could otherwise be used to prevent illness. Studies carried out at the Common Cold Unit at Oxford University showed that

THE THREE PHASES OF STRESS

Researchers have found that the body uses energy in three sequential phases when faced with a stressful situation. The third phase, worrying about a recent experience, can help you better recognize danger and prevent a similar situation in the future. However, this stage is very draining if you cannot turn off the stress and relax. Try to review the crisis calmly and understand that the danger has passed and you are safe.

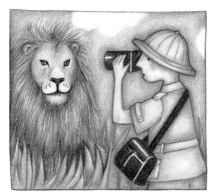

PREPARING ENERGY
In phase one you ready yourself, harnessing energy reserves. You sense the danger and your body is preparing for a "fight or flight" reaction.

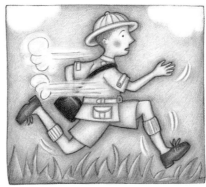

UTILIZING ENERGY
In phase two you are using your energy reserves. Your body is working to its full potential to help you get through the situation.

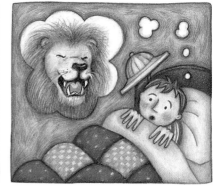

DRAINING ENERGY
In phase three stress continues and drains your energy for no purpose. You may be out of danger but your body and mind cannot calm down.

Clear Your Mind with

Standing Meditation

The most important and widely practiced form of chi kung is standing meditation. It aims to develop better alignment and balance, stronger legs and waist, deeper respiration, body awareness, and a tranquil mind.

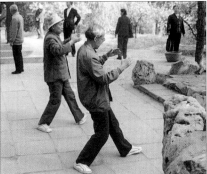

DAILY BREAK
Many Chinese people practice chi kung every day for health, often outdoors in squares or parks.

Practice this exercise at first for 5 minutes each day, spending equal amounts of time in each position. After a week, increase the time to 15 minutes a day; after three weeks you should be able to meditate for 20 to 40 minutes at a time. Stand with your feet a little more than hip width apart and knees slightly bent. Try to achieve a natural alignment of the spine, free from tension. It can help to imagine a thread pulling up from the base of your neck through the top of your head. Begin the exercise with both arms relaxed and slightly in front of your body.

SIMPLE STANDING MEDITATION

Spend a minute or two concentrating your attention on your body. Begin by focusing on your feet and then work your way up through each part of the body, paying particular attention to the spine. Relax and free up any tension, feeling the contact of your feet with the floor.

Eyes should be open and relaxed.

Arms should be in a rounded position in front of you.

Feet should be a little more than hip width apart.

1 *Hold your hands out in front of your abdomen, with both palms facing toward your body as if embracing a large, lightweight ball. Inhale slowly and move your hands upward to your waistline, palms facing the body. Hold the position for a few seconds.*

Be aware of whatever presents itself in your consciousness, giving yourself permission to feel or think anything that you want.

Hands may be raised to your head, but not above.

Breathing should be natural and relaxed and supported by the diaphragm.

2 *Raise your hands farther up your body while inhaling, bringing them in toward your head and gently turning your palms around to face forward. Hold for a few seconds, then slowly start to exhale and work your arms and hands down in front of you, palms facing your body. Repeat the whole exercise several times.*

people who had suffered negative emotions during the previous six months and whose coping skills were poor were more likely to develop colds than those who had good coping skills for negative emotions. In addition, the incidence of colds was significantly higher in those who were introverted, indicating that people who can call on a good support group are better able to handle the difficult emotions such experiences generate than those who hold them inside.

Learning to use your energy wisely will enable you to build a reserve for emergencies. If you learn to recognize your physical and emotional thresholds, you can then take preventative actions before you deplete your energy reserves.

CHOOSING YOUR EMOTIONS

Most negative emotions and thoughts can be turned into positive ones by rechanneling energies into good actions. Some psychologists believe that we choose the emotions we experience. When we reach our threshold of endurance—which we ourselves set—we permit ourselves to "go over the edge" and express our frustration. Where we set these limits can be reasonable, that is, at a level where most people would be inclined to set them, or unreasonable, making our reactions extreme or inappropriate or brought about by irrational thinking.

How you react to a situation is up to you. If you don't like your job, find another one. If this is not possible, you can at least try to make adjustments from within; have a talk with your boss, suggest changes in procedures, or request a transfer to another department. It is important to remember that you always have options.

Some negative emotions, when viewed from another perspective, can become positive. Anger does not have to be negative; it can serve as a trigger to do something constructive about the situation that is aggravating you. Envy can be transformed into admiration and become an inspiration. Anxiety can help you recognize situations in which you need to learn better coping skills.

Feeling empowered is highly energizing and motivating. The elation you get from achieving something positive cancels out

---

A FRIEND IN NEED

When friends or relatives are at a low ebb and perhaps do not know where to turn—or even know why they are feeling so unhappy—you can give invaluable comfort. Even if you cannot help in practical ways, just listening allows the other person to share his or her anxieties and reduce stress. If you need support, do not be afraid to ask friends or family for help. They can bring new perspectives to a problem.

Listening is the most helpful thing you can do. Try to empathize with the person and attempt to understand what has triggered such unhappiness.

Help if you can. Perhaps you can offer a practical solution or the address of a professional organization that can provide assistance. Make sure that the person wants you to help! Sometimes it is better just to listen.

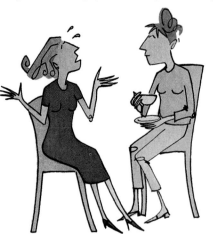

ASK QUESTIONS
After listening, try to ask questions that will help the other person focus on the problem. It may reveal aspects that had not previously been considered and provide an opportunity to see the problem from a different angle.

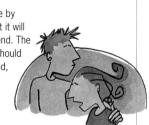

Comfort and console by telling the person that it will all be all right in the end. The value of comforting should not be underestimated, although it should be backed up with practical help whenever possible.

Support is important. Few crises disappear overnight, and emotional problems are no exception. Your role as friend is to provide long-term support. Visit and phone regularly. Be the type of friend you would want for yourself.

Do not pass judgment, whatever the problem is, and avoid criticism. Professional counselors aim to reveal to sufferers ways in which they can help themselves. They rarely offer their own opinions; neither should you.

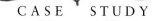
An Irritable Mother

Emotional problems can seriously drain energy, especially if they are ignored or repressed. In such circumstances some people express their pent-up feelings through bitterness or anger. Taking time to identify and acknowledge the causes of distress and talking these over with family, a counselor, or close friends can help a person get through difficult times.

Roselyn is a fulltime mother with two sons in grade school. Her husband has recently been promoted and often spends time away on business, leaving her to look after the boys on her own. Her mother died unexpectedly last year of leukemia, and Roselyn has found herself growing stoical about life, not admitting that her emotions are getting her down. She has been experiencing a general loss of energy and difficulties in leaving the house. She is snapping at the children and her husband, blaming his absence for all her problems. She went to see her doctor and had a series of tests for fatigue disorders, but no specific cause could be determined. Her doctor suggested that she go to see a counselor.

WHAT SHOULD ROSELYN DO?

Roselyn should go to a counselor, who will talk with her about her life and lifestyle and how she feels about her family. Counseling could help Roselyn to root out the underlying cause of her irritability and unhappiness by allowing her to talk freely about her emotions and uncover deeper problems and anxieties. Facing her mother's death and allowing time for proper grieving should be a priority. Rather than snapping at her family, she must talk calmly to them about her needs, and they in turn should arrange to give her time and space to recover. The doctor may also prescribe a short course of antidepressants to help Roselyn cope with her unstable emotions.

Action Plan

LIFESTYLE
Make time for self. Keeping too busy to face problems only allows them to build up inside.

DEPRESSION
Talk to a counselor who can help to identify and resolve the underlying causes of depression. Understanding and facing emotions is the first step to emotional health.

FAMILY
Talk to family and friends about worries and grief. Recognize that irritability and anger are counter-productive means of expression.

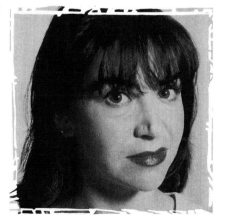

FAMILY
Family problems can build up if you do not openly discuss issues as they arise.

LIFESTYLE
Keeping going without proper rest can seriously damage your emotional and physical health.

DEPRESSION
Depression can drain energy and create emotional crises and other difficulties.

HOW THINGS TURNED OUT FOR ROSELYN

Roselyn's counseling helped her to accept the toll her mother's death was taking on her emotional and physical health. She became aware that she had alienated her husband as a result of his being away, and they spent time restoring their relationship. He adjusted his work schedule so that he could spend more time at home. She joined a local chi kung class, which helped her to relax and restore her emotional and physical energy.

ORGANIZE AND PRIORITIZE

Whether at work or in your personal life, learning to organize and prioritize clears away confusion and allows you to be more efficient.

▶ *Keep up-to-date with your filing so you know where everything is and when it needs attention.*

▶ *Keep a wall calendar and diary. Look at them every day to see what you have to do.*

▶ *Keep a list. Write down everything you need to do and check off those you have done.*

▶ *Prioritize your list. Categorize entries, marking those that are urgent.*

▶ *Don't use delaying tactics. Phone people you have to phone and leave personal calls for later.*

▶ *Learn how to say "no." Recognize your limits and don't take on what you can't do.*

▶ *Keep a set of accounts so you can see how much you are spending and how much you have.*

▶ *Learn to delegate. You do not have to do everything yourself.*

*KEEPING IN TOUCH
Friendships are among the most rewarding parts of our lives, supporting us through the bad times and giving us another point of view.*

negative feelings and beliefs that can be harmful. Taking charge of your life can bring a great boost to your energy.

YOUR SUPPORT MECHANISMS

Even the most self-sufficient of us can recognize the positive help that others can provide. There are times when it is unwise to fight battles on your own, and recognizing when you need help from friends or a counselor or could use spiritual guidance will help you through your problems.

Spiritual guidance

In times of emotional distress, many people feel a need for spiritual or religious support. Irrespective of religious doctrine, most leaders of religious groups are trained in supporting those who are going through a crisis. Religious beliefs can be very comforting in times of emotional upset, when the world ceases to make any sense. Many alternative therapies offer different spiritual philosophies that can also refresh your outlook and help you to view the world from a different and healthier angle.

Friendship

One of the greatest support systems you have is your friends, and because they are likely to be familiar with your circumstances, they may be able to offer useful and supportive advice. However, you should choose a confidant wisely. Select someone who will listen, help, and, above all, be able to keep a confidence. This may be a person other than your best friend or partner; it can often be better to talk to someone who is not involved and can see your problems from an objective standpoint.

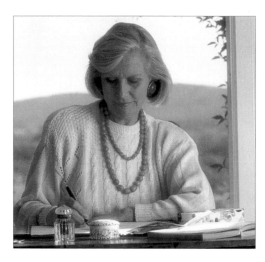

CHANGE YOUR LIFE

Change begets change. If you alter one thing in your life, you will find that other things change around it, providing you with a new direction and focus. Change is renewing and replenishing, providing you with the opportunity to fulfill yourself in new ways. Change can also be daunting, but if you make changes gradually, they will seem less intimidating.

Be positive about change. Pursue new interests or hobbies that provide you with mental and/or physical stimulation. Join a gym, a dance class, or an evening course. Become a volunteer for a charity; help yourself through helping others.

Don't forget to challenge your brain, particularly if you do not work or are retired. Learn a new language, study literature or history, join a reading group, or become an expert in something that interests you.

Counseling

Sometimes problems are deeply rooted or very complex and require the skills of a professional counselor. Such people are trained to ask questions and listen to you, helping you to sort out your own problems rather than making any judgments or diagnoses for you or giving advice. In this way counseling can give you insight into your feelings and empower you to solve your own problems. With the guidance of a counselor, you may be able to resolve inner conflicts and find practical solutions. If you feel that counseling could be useful for you, ask your doctor to refer you to someone who is trained to help with the kind of difficulty you are experiencing.

Energizing therapies

There are alternative therapies that can help you revitalize your energy channels, removing stresses and pressures and releasing unwanted tension. Many of these rely on Eastern holistic philosophies (see page 48), which view energy as a universal force that flows through your body. Therapies such as t'ai chi, chi kung, Reiki, and shiatsu aim to rebalance your energy, allowing your natural restorative forces to work freely.

CHAPTER 6

SERIOUS CONDITIONS AND ILLNESSES

If you are lacking in energy for a prolonged period, you may have a serious underlying condition. Conventional tests can identify a specific illness, and various treatments can help counter both the ailment and the lack of energy. Some energy disorders, however, benefit most from a holistic approach that involves diet, exercise, and stress reduction.

CONSULTING YOUR DOCTOR

Lack of energy is commonly associated with an underlying medical condition. Locating and treating a debilitating condition can restore your vitality, as well as your health.

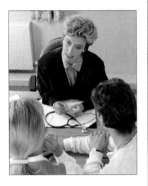

GO PREPARED
Before visiting a doctor, make a brief list of your symptoms and bodily changes so you do not forget to mention something during the consultation that may help with your diagnosis.

Most people feel tired and lacking in energy from time to time, and determining the cause can be difficult. You may be just having a bad day or experiencing a minor illness. However, if fatigue has been nagging and persistent for a few weeks or more, it's time to consider if recent circumstances in your life are at fault or if there may be a more serious problem to consider. Have you been eating properly, exercising regularly, getting sufficient sleep? If you cannot locate a possible cause for your fatigue, such as a cold or unusual stress, you should make an appointment with your primary care physician.

VISITING YOUR DOCTOR
Although there are many possible causes for fatigue—physical, emotional, and/or psychological—physical disorders are generally the easiest to diagnose and treat, and they are frequently the problem. In one study an American physician, Dr. John D. Morrison, reviewed the cases of 176 patients who had chronic fatigue. He found that 69 of the them, or about 40 percent, were experiencing minor or serious physical problems, including viral infections, a heart or lung disorder, arthritis, or nutritional deficiencies. In addition, 21 patients were suffering from combined physical and psychological

WHAT CAN MEDICAL TESTS TELL YOU?

A number of tests may be carried out initially, including a general physical examination and blood and urine analyses, which can indicate possible problem areas. Further tests may be done to locate more specific problems. You may find yourself referred to a specialist or hospital department for further tests and treatment.

FULL EXAMINATION
A thorough examination usually includes assessing the condition of your skin, hair, nails, tongue, eyes, ears, chest, abdomen, lymph glands, nervous system, heart, lung function, blood circulation, and reproductive health.

▶ **NUTRITIONAL TESTS**
The blood can be tested for a range of nutrient deficiencies, including iron, vitamin B_{12}, folic acid, other B vitamins, magnesium, and zinc.

▶ **OTHER BLOOD TESTS**
With certain blood tests the numbers and shapes of blood cells are examined to identify infections or diseases like sickle cell anemia.

▶ **URINE TEST**
A quick and easy urine test can show up kidney, bladder, and urethral disorders, as well as low blood sugar levels and diabetes.

▶ **INFECTION TESTS**
Immunoglobulin tests can monitor antibody levels and indicate hidden infections.

▶ **THYROID TEST**
If a patient has energy problems, the levels of thyroid hormones in the blood are measured to find any imbalances.

difficulties. In 72 other cases, psychological problems alone were the primary cause of chronic fatigue. Studies by other researchers have revealed that blood abnormalities can play a major role in fatigue, and thyroid disorders are a common cause of complaints.

Before you visit your doctor, make a note of any physical changes that have occurred. Has your weight inexplicably gone up or down? Have you had any fever or night sweats? Are you often constipated? Have you experienced double vision or ringing in the ears? Has your appetite changed?

If your doctor does not find any apparent physical problems that are causing lack of energy, there is a chance that it is psychological. Medical experts believe that some fatigue patients are suffering from a psychosomatic reaction to a major emotional upheaval, such as the death of a loved one or pressure to achieve more than they are capable of. In these cases a doctor may recommend psychotherapy. However, many psychological problems can themselves be the result of physical disorders and must not be assumed to be the only or primary cause of fatigue. The interaction between the mind and body can have a subtle but significant impact on the whole system.

Many prescription and over-the-counter medicines have toxic side effects that can drain energy; ask your doctor or druggist if this is a possibility. The action may be indirect. For instance, some medications interfere with the absorption of certain nutrients or cause them to be excreted. Diuretics are an example of the latter; they can drain potassium and magnesium from the body.

WHAT MAY BE CAUSING YOUR FATIGUE

Fatigue is the symptom of a number of disorders. One of the most difficult tasks that a physician faces is finding which single factor or combination of factors is causing a lack of energy. It is important to go to your doctor if you suffer from any of the symptoms listed below recurrently or for a prolonged period. The table is a general guide only and is no substitute for a doctor's examination.

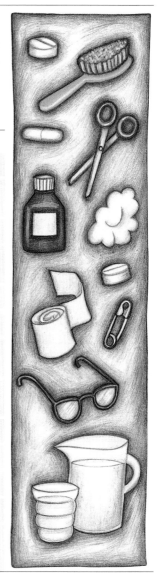

SYMPTOMS	POSSIBLE CAUSES
Have you experienced tiredness just recently?	Infection
Do you feel particularly tired when getting up in the morning?	Hypoglycemia; insomnia, apnea, or other sleeping disorders
Do you feel tiredness with a headache or dizziness?	High or low blood pressure; hypoglycemia
Do you have tiredness associated with digestive troubles?	Enzyme deficiency; disturbed flora in the gut
Do you feel ill if you miss a meal?	Hypoglycemia
Is your tongue red, sore, or fissured?	Anemia
Have you suffered from a loss of hair on your head, skin dryness, or constant chilliness?	Thyroid gland deficiency
Have you noticed a deterioration of eyesight, a great thirst, or poor wound healing?	Diabetes; nutritional deficiency
Do you get breathless easily?	Heart or lung problems
Have you had a recent head injury?	Shock to the nervous system
Do you bruise easily?	Anemia; nutritional deficiency
Do you have swelling of the ankles and feet?	Heart or circulation disorder
Have you been suffering from recurrent infections?	Depression of immune system; diabetes; thyroid deficiency

High or Low Blood Pressure

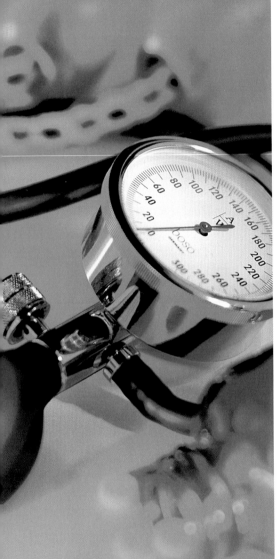

High blood pressure, very common in North America, can lead to heart disease and stroke if left untreated. Mildly low blood pressure is not generally a reason for concern unless it causes a person to faint and sustain an injury.

THE PROBLEM

Blood pressure is an indication of the power of the heartbeat and the amount of resistance in the blood circulation. A reasonable pressure must be sustained to ensure that sufficient blood reaches the brain and limbs. But if the pressure falls dramatically low or is consistently too high, physical disorders ensue.

Blood pressure is recorded as two numbers that measure the pressure when a cuff is tightened around the arm to stop blood flow, then gradually released. The higher figure (systolic) represents the pressure during the heart's contraction phase; the lower figure (diastolic) measures the relaxation phase.

Normal blood pressure for an adult is below 140/85; it is slightly lower in children and a little higher in the elderly. Blood pressure varies a bit according to activity, but if it remains consistently high, it is known as hypertension. At the other end of the scale is hypotension, indicated by a systolic pressure below 100.

High blood pressure may be caused by a disease of the heart, kidneys, lungs, liver, or blood vessels. In the majority of cases, however, there is no apparent cause, and this is known as essential hypertension. Persistent high blood pressure can be a serious threat to health, with a greater risk of stroke or heart attack.

Low blood pressure is sometimes signaled by light-headedness when changing position quickly and coldness of the extremities. It can be caused by medication for high blood pressure or may indicate a weakness of the adrenal glands, anemia, or generally poor nourishment. A sudden dramatic drop in blood pressure, or clinical shock, usually results from injury or serious disease and is a life-threatening condition that requires emergency aid.

Both high and low blood pressure may be responsible for tiredness but rarely show obvious symptoms; most often they are discovered when blood pressure is tested during a routine medical examination. Once detected, high blood pressure should be monitored regularly and regulated with professional guidance on diet and lifestyle, supported by medications when necessary.

BLOOD PRESSURE FACTORS

Several factors, especially when combined, are thought to contribute to hypertension; they include

► *Being overweight*

► *Consuming too much salt, sugar, caffeine, and/or alcohol*

► *Smoking*

► *Intensely competitive personality*

► *Prolonged stress*

► *Toxemia of pregnancy or use of oral contraceptives*

► *A lack of regular exercise*

SYMPTOMS

Of low blood pressure

► Light-headedness or dizziness upon standing

► Frequent fainting spells

► Cold extremities

► Fatigue

Of high blood pressure

► General ill health, including fatigue

► Headaches

► Palpitations

DIETARY MEASURES

Dietary modifications form the cornerstone of hypertension management. Some cases improve simply with a reduction in weight. For anyone who is overweight, losing just 5 to 10 pounds can have a dramatic impact on blood pressure.

▶ **Reduce salt.**
High salt intake contributes to high blood pressure in some individuals. Such people need to limit other sources of sodium as well.

▶ **Increase potassium and calcium.**
Foods that are rich in potassium—many fruits, vegetables, as well as legumes—help the body to regulate sodium. Calcium also has a beneficial effect on blood pressure in people who are salt sensitive.

▶ **Cut down on saturated fat.**
Saturated fat, the kind prevalent in meat and dairy products, can lead to a buildup of fatty deposits in the arteries and restrict blood flow.

▶ **Avoid stimulants.**
Both caffeine and nicotine cause a temporary increase in blood pressure.

▶ **Eat more fish and/or flaxseed oil.**
The omega-3 fatty acids present in oily fish and flaxseeds have been shown to reduce blood pressure.

Complementary approaches

For hypertension, a naturopath may recommend fresh juices or lacto-fermented juices as good sources of potassium and magnesium, which help balance blood pressure. Short fasts with juices and raw-food dietary regimens under naturopathic supervision can be effective in lowering blood pressure. In one trial, a diet of raw fruits and vegetables was found to be as effective as conventional drugs in reducing blood pressure. Supplements of vitamins C and E, also magnesium, garlic, and coenzyme Q10, have benefited many people who have hypertension.

HERBAL TREATMENT

An extract of hawthorn (*Crataegus oxyacantha*) is reputed to restore blood pressure balance in cases of either hypertension or hypotension. Herbs with blood-pressure-lowering properties include garlic (*Allium sativum*) and skullcap (*Scutellaria lateriflora*). Mild herbal diuretics, which stimulate excretion of excess sodium, are corn silk and dandelion, taken as teas or extracts.

People who have low blood pressure tend to be easily fatigued. Suitable herbal remedies may help compensate for these susceptibilities. In particular, tonic herbs may be suggested to sustain the cardiac output and support the tone of blood vessels, as well as glands such as the adrenals. Ginseng (*Panax ginseng*) and prickly ash (*Xanthoxylum americanum*) are herbs that are often considered.

ACUPRESSURE POINTS

The powerful relaxation effects of acupressure are believed to account for its success in treating high blood pressure. This traditional Chinese technique of rebalancing energy through pressure relieves stress and enhances well-being by opening the energy channels at specific points where blockages occur. Apply firm but gentle pressure to the following acupressure points, using a fingertip or thumb, for two or three minutes at a time. You may also use dispersed pressure by gently massaging the area.

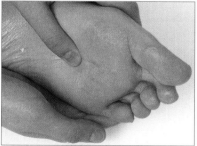

KIDNEY 1
This is on the bottom of the foot, in the central depression one-third of the way between the toes and the heel.

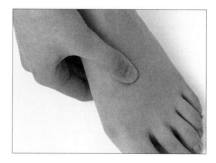

LIVER 3
This point is on the top of the foot, in the angle between the long bones leading to the first and second toes.

HYDROTHERAPY

Several hydrotherapy techniques can help increase circulation that may be sluggish due to low blood pressure or other conditions.

▶ *Turn your morning shower cold for a few seconds before you get out. This stimulates the blood to circulate faster and is particularly good for the skin and hair.*

▶ *Use alternate hot and cold foot baths to encourage better blood flow in the arteries. Spend a few minutes in each before you change.*

▶ *Place an ice pack or a cold, damp washcloth against the back of your neck; it will force the blood to pump faster around your body.*

▶ *Go for a swim. Even if you are not a strong swimmer, the activity is great for moderating blood pressure, as well as benefiting all-round health. Do stretching exercises in the water to keep flexible.*

Heart and Artery Diseases

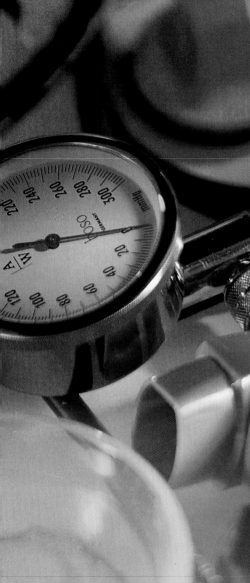

Heart and artery diseases, which kill more than 1¼ million North Americans annually, severely restrict the lives of many people, draining energy and preventing normal activity. They can often be prevented with simple changes in diet and lifestyle.

THE PROBLEM

Heart and artery diseases are often caused by fatty deposits, or plaques, that build up on the walls of the arteries, resulting in narrowing and eventually blockage—a condition known as atherosclerosis. The heart needs a constant supply of oxygen, glucose, and other nutrients, which it receives through its own network of blood vessels called coronary arteries. If these arteries become narrowed by fatty plaques, the blood flow to the heart muscle is restricted, and the heart can no longer cope with exertion like walking upstairs. Strenuous physical effort may cause severe chest pain—a condition called angina pectoris, which can limit a sufferer's ability to lead a normal life.

Once a coronary artery is blocked completely, the part of the heart that it nourishes dies, causing intense pain and other symptoms of a heart attack, although some heart attacks are painless and detected only later with an electrocardiogram. The severity of a heart attack depends on the amount of heart muscle damaged, but it is always serious and often fatal, causing half a million deaths a year in the United States alone.

AGE CONCERN
As you grow older, the chances of suffering from a heart or an artery disorder increase greatly. Regular exercise and a healthful dietary regimen can help to lower the risk.

SYMPTOMS

▶ Tiredness during and after physical exertion

▶ General fatigue

▶ Pains in the chest

▶ Irregular heartbeat or heart palpitations

▶ Blueness of the skin caused by a lack of oxygen in the blood

▶ A feeling of faintness after physical exertion

CAUSES OF HEART AND ARTERY DISEASES

The risk of developing heart disease is increased by several factors; the ones listed here can be controlled.

▶ *A diet high in naturally saturated and hydrogenated fats, found in such foods as meat, dairy products, and fried foods*

▶ *High levels of cholesterol, particularly the LDL form*

▶ *Being overweight*

▶ *Smoking*

▶ *Drinking too much alcohol*

▶ *An inactive lifestyle*

▶ *A diet too high in iron*

▶ *High blood pressure*

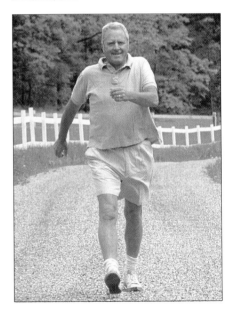

DEALING WITH A HEART ATTACK

Knowing what to do if you or someone near you has a heart attack can save a life. The symptoms often start as a mild ache in the chest that may be confused with indigestion. This commonly turns into moderate or severe pain in the center of the chest that radiates to the neck, shoulders, jaw, arms, or back. It is often accompanied by dizziness, sweating, clamminess, nausea, shallow and rapid breathing, and sometimes a sense of impending danger.

Not every symptom is always present. In some cases symptoms subside and return later. Studies show that half of heart attack victims wait more than two hours before getting help—a delay that can prove fatal.

The first priority in a heart attack is to dial 911 and ask for an ambulance. Loosen the patient's clothing and ease him or her into a half-sitting position, with head fully supported and knees bent to minimize strain on the heart. If the person suffers from angina, he or she may have glyceryl trinitrate (GTN) as tablets or inhaler. Give one tablet or two puffs of the inhaler. If pain persists and the sufferer is fully conscious, provide an aspirin tablet to chew slowly or swallow without water. If the patient loses consciousness place in the recovery position. Should breathing stop, apply cardiopulmonary resuscitation if you have learned the technique.

FOOD SUPPLEMENTS

Antioxidants, such as vitamins C and E and the mineral selenium, have proved effective in helping prevent heart and artery disease when increased in the diet and/or taken as supplements. In several studies an increase in antioxidants reduced the risk of heart disease by up to 40 percent in men and 25 percent in women. Supplements that have improved heart function in cases of congestive heart failure, mitral valve prolapse, and obstructive damage include magnesium and coenzyme Q10 (see page 109). Supplements should be taken only with the supervision of a doctor for optimal results.

REDUCING THE RISK OF HEART AND ARTERY DISEASES

Diet and lifestyle are the main underlying causes of heart and artery diseases. Positive changes in these can go a long way toward reducing the risk of heart attack. They can also make a significant difference to general health and energy.

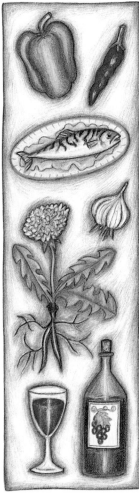

EAT MORE FRUITS AND VEGETABLES

Eat plenty of brightly colored fruits and vegetables, which contain antioxidants, including beta carotene and vitamin C. These protect the heart against free radicals—unstable molecules produced by metabolic processes and pollution—which encourage fat buildup.

EAT MORE FIBER

Soluble fiber, found in fruits, vegetables, legumes, and oat bran, reduces blood cholesterol levels.

EAT OILY FISH

Include plenty of oily fish, such as salmon and tuna, in your diet. These types of fish contain omega-3 fatty acids, which can strengthen the heart, lower blood pressure, and lower blood cholesterol levels.

MANAGE STRESS

Control your stress levels. Stress leads to raised blood pressure and increases the risk of heart and artery diseases. Relaxation exercises can help.

TAKE AN ASPIRIN

Consider taking half an aspirin tablet each day to reduce the stickiness of the blood platelets and prevent blood clots. Discuss this with your doctor.

KEEP ACTIVE

An inactive lifestyle is a major cause of heart disease. Stay active and, in particular, regularly do aerobic exercise, such as brisk walking, running, cycling, or swimming, for 20 to 30 minutes three times a week. This strengthens heart muscle and inhibits fat buildup.

CONSIDER HORMONE REPLACEMENT

If you are postmenopausal, consider hormone replacement therapy (HRT) to help protect against heart disease.

SPICE UP YOUR LIFE

Include more fresh ginger and chili peppers in the diet. Ginger helps lower cholesterol and blood pressure and reduces the risk of clotting. Chili peppers may prevent blood clots that can lead to a heart attack or stroke.

MODERATE DRINKING

Excessive alcohol damages heart muscle. In moderation drinking, especially red wine, can be beneficial because it raises levels of protective high-density lipoproteins.

TRY HERBAL REMEDIES

Ginkgo biloba increases blood flow to the heart and extremities. Garlic lowers cholesterol levels and blood pressure and inhibits the tendency of blood to clot.

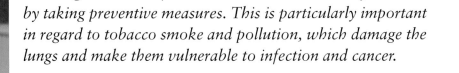

Lung Disorders

The lungs are at risk from various diseases that may be avoided by taking preventive measures. This is particularly important in regard to tobacco smoke and pollution, which damage the lungs and make them vulnerable to infection and cancer.

THE PROBLEMS

As you breathe, your lungs take in particles, such as dust, fumes, micro-organisms, and allergens, along with the air. As a result, the lungs are under constant threat from toxic substances and diseases. In cases of congestive heart failure, the lungs can also be affected by the buildup of fluid in the lungs.

Infection is the most common lung disorder. A severe infection can lead to acute bronchitis—inflammation of the airways (bronchi) that branch off the windpipe. When a serious viral or bacterial infection spreads to the surrounding lung tissue, it causes pneumonia. If it spreads to the membranes (pleura) that line and surround the lungs, it causes pleurisy. Both conditions require urgent medical attention.

Acute bronchitis disappears once an infection is over. But chronic bronchitis can last indefinitely. It is usually caused by cigarette smoking, polluted air, or exposure to dust or fumes at work, any of which irritate the bronchi. Chronic bronchitis that causes extensive damage to lung tissue can result in emphysema. This is a serious, incurable condition in which the groups of air sacs (alveoli) that absorb oxygen break down, making breathing extremely difficult.

Asthma often results from an allergy—to airborne particles, such as house dust, pollen, pet hairs and feathers, and chemical sprays, or to

CAUSES OF LUNG PROBLEMS

Common causes of lung disorders are infections, arterial problems, and airborne pollutants. Conditions with air pollution are made worse by poor ventilation, such as in airplanes and high-rise buildings.

▶ *Viral or bacterial infection*

▶ *Air pollutants, such as dust, soot, and vehicle exhaust fumes*

▶ *Airborne allergens, such as pollen and dust mites*

▶ *Inhaling of tobacco smoke or other drugs directly*

▶ *Smoky atmospheres, for example, in bars*

certain foods. It causes contraction of the muscles of the bronchi and increased production of mucus in the lungs. Asthma is usually chronic, occurring as periodic attacks. Patients need to manage the condition by avoiding known irritants and using inhalant drugs to clear congestion.

Certain jobs carry a risk of occupational lung disorders, and it is important for people in these occupations to take precautions. Pneumoconiosis can develop from coal dust, asbestosis from asbestos fibers, silicosis from stone dust, and byssinosis from textile fibers. These can lead to emphysema and, along with smoking, are also common

SYMPTOMS

▶ Persistent cough with thick yellow, green, or gray phlegm

▶ Persistent coughing, wheezing, or shortness of breath

▶ Difficulty breathing

▶ Blood in the phlegm

▶ Chest pain

▶ A blue tinge to the skin

▶ A high temperature or chills

▶ Swollen legs

AVOIDING LUNG DISORDERS

The lungs become irritated by atmospheres that are constantly very wet because molds develop. Living in a damp home raises the risk of developing chronic bronchitis. It is important to deal with dampness by using dehumidifiers and making sure that you have good ventilation.

The very dry, dusty atmospheres created by central heating and air conditioning systems in homes and offices can also irritate the lining of the lungs and increase the risk of colds, flu, coughs, and asthma. Dry air also thickens mucus, making it more difficult to expel. You can improve air quality by providing adequate ventilation and by using a humidifier or placing bowls of water near heaters to humidify the air.

Asthma sufferers need to identify allergens and avoid them whenever possible. Mold spores, house dust, and animal dander are common culprits. Regular cleaning prevents a buildup of these irritants, and some vacuum cleaners now have special filters that capture a high percentage of them and prevent them from recirculating in the air. Special filters are available as well that filter out air pollutants in a room. Asthma sufferers also need to avoid exercising outdoors when pollen counts are high.

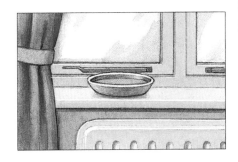

HUMIDIFIER
Keeping the atmosphere of a room moist can help to ease or prevent lung problems. A dish of water on a radiator is an inexpensive and easy alternative to a humidifier for moisturizing air.

SUPPLEMENTS

Supplements may be taken, with the supervision of a doctor or nutritionist, to improve immunity and prevent lung disorders when sufficient amounts are not obtained from food (see below). The antioxidant vitamins, A, C, and E, are especially important.

▶ *Vitamin A is quickly destroyed by cigarette smoke and atmospheric pollution, so supplements may be helpful for some people. Too much of this vitamin is harmful, however; the recommended daily dosage should not be greatly exceeded.*

▶ *During the winter or when you have an active infection, take 500 mg of vitamin C twice a day.*

▶ *Vitamin E helps to reduce the inflammation of lung infection.*

▶ *Zinc supplements aid the immune system. Sucking a zinc lozenge at regular intervals can also help to prevent a viral infection.*

TREATING LUNG DISORDERS

For many lung disorders, avoiding the underlying causes—cigarette smoke, polluted air, or specific allergens—is the only realistic approach. Most infections will run their course naturally. Resting in relatively dry, warm conditions and eating healthfully are usually sufficient treatment. More serious infections require medical attention.

Cough medicines are of limited use. They are available in three basic types: expectorants, which loosen the mucus of a chesty cough so that it can be more easily expelled, cough suppressants, which soothe dry, irritating coughs, and a combination of these two. A cough suppressant should not be taken for a chesty cough because it can cause mucus to build up in the lungs and may lead to a more serious lung disorder. An effective measure for loosening the mucus and opening the airways is steam inhalation. Pour hot water into a bowl and inhale the vapor. You can add a few drops of menthol, eucalyptus, or peppermint oil to enhance the effectiveness.

Regular aerobic exercise helps strengthen lungs and reduce the risk of lung disorders. Brisk walking, cycling, jogging, or swimming for at least 20 minutes three times a week can be effective. Even people with chronic bronchitis find that regular exercise improves lung function and reduces feelings of breathlessness. Start with a few minutes of activity and build up as you feel stronger. Stop at once if you are very breathless or have chest pains. Lung capacity can also be improved by regular deep-breathing exercises, drawing air from the abdomen rather than taking rapid, shallow breaths.

NUTRITIONAL ADVICE

Vitamins C and A are vital for a healthy immune system and to protect delicate lung tissue from the cellular damage caused by free radicals, unstable molecules that are released when the body burns oxygen. They are also crucial for repairing cells, especially the mucous lining of the lungs.

Vitamin C is plentiful in kiwi and citrus fruits, berries, peppers, broccoli, potatoes, and many other vegetables. Vitamin A is easily obtained from orange and yellow fruits and vegetables and green leafy ones like spinach. It is also found in liver, fish, and fortified milk.

Intake of the refined sugar used in candies, cakes, cookies, and soft drinks should be limited because it depresses the immune system.

Anemia

Many people suffer from anemia, which reduces the body's ability to produce energy and leads to deep and prolonged fatigue. Making sure that you get the right nutrients can prevent anemia and make up deficiencies in mild cases.

THE PROBLEM

If you are persistently tired, one of the first things your doctor may do is test your blood for anemia—a deficiency of red blood corpuscles or the hemoglobin they carry. Anemia diminishes the ability of the blood to carry oxygen to all the body tissues, thus starving them. Symptoms of mild anemia include pallor, fatigue, lethargy, brittle, spoon-shaped nails, and headaches; more severe cases are marked by difficulty breathing, dizziness, and cardiac arrhythmia.

There are many types of anemia, some of them caused by metabolic defects, certain medications, or environmental toxins. However, the most common forms are caused by a deficiency of the nutrients needed for the formation of hemoglobin, in particular iron but also vitamin B_{12} and folic acid. (Deficiency of B_{12} is known as "pernicious anemia.")

The people most at risk for iron deficiency are women who bleed heavily during their menstrual periods, children under age two who obtain most of their nourishment from milk, pregnant women, vegetarians, people with bleeding ulcers, alcoholics, and the elderly. Surgical patients and accident victims who hemorrhage are also at risk.

An accurate diagnosis of anemia requires blood analysis, starting with a complete blood count in which the various cells in a specific amount of blood are counted under a micro-

scope and examined for abnormalities in their shape, size, color, and distribution. When iron is deficient, the red blood cells are very small; they become large with deficiencies of folic acid or vitamin B_{12}.

CAUSES OF ANEMIA

The most common causes of anemia are deficiencies of certain nutrients, but there can be other factors.

▶ *Insufficient iron or vitamin B_{12} or folic acid in the diet*
▶ *Inability to absorb some nutrients*
▶ *A large or steady loss of blood*
▶ *Autoimmune disease in which red blood cells are destroyed*
▶ *Inability of bone marrow to make enough red blood cells*

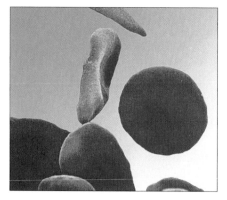

ANEMIC BLOOD CELLS
Red blood cells obtain their color from hemoglobin, an iron-rich protein that carries oxygen. Insufficient iron is the most prevalent cause of anemia.

SYMPTOMS

▶ Tiredness and lethargy
▶ Pale complexion, sometimes with a green or blue tinge
▶ Recurring headaches
▶ Poor skin, hair, and nail condition
▶ Loss of appetite
▶ Breathlessness after physical exertion
▶ Dizziness and inability to concentrate
▶ Difficulty breathing

DIETARY MEASURES

Several nutrients are essential for the formation of healthy red blood cells. Iron, copper, and vitamins C, B_{12}, and folic acid all play an important role.

The richest sources of iron are red meat, liver, seafood, and poultry, all of which contain heme iron, the most readily absorbed form. Whole grains; legumes, especially soybeans; dried prunes and apricots; broccoli, beet greens, and other leafy greens; and blackstrap molasses are rich in non-heme iron, a form that is less easily utilized but valuable nonetheless. Absorption of nonheme iron is enhanced by the presence of vitamin C.

Although spinach has a high iron content, it also contains oxalic acid, which binds with iron and limits its absorption. Another compound that inhibits iron absorption is phytate, found in cereal brans (see page 106).

A number of the foods listed above are also good sources of other nutrients needed for blood forma-tion, including copper, folic acid, and vitamin B_{12}. In addition, some bread, cereal products, and soy products are fortified with iron, folic acid, and vitamin B_{12}. These foods can be beneficial especially to vegetarians. Cooking in iron utensils is another way to obtain iron in the diet.

Vegetables that have been through a lacto-fermentation process or have been made into a juice are reputedly good for blood disorders because they are easier to absorb. The process breaks down the indigestible cellulose component, making the food an excellent source of nutrients.

Some disorders can affect the ability of the intestines to produce a substance called intrinsic factor, which is necessary for the absorption of vitamin B_{12}. Insufficient hydro-chloric acid in the stomach can have the same effect, and there may be a need in such cases to provide supple-ments (see box, right).

SUPPLEMENTS

The dietary measures recommended to the left will usually prevent anemia and can correct it in mild cases. For anemia that is more severe, supple-ments may be needed but should be taken under the supervision of a doc-tor or nutritionist. Iron, in particular, can be toxic in high doses.

▶ *Iron deficiency is the primary cause of anemia, and supplements may be needed to correct it. These are available in both heme and nonheme forms, of which the heme is more easily absorbed.*

▶ *Vitamin C improves the uptake of iron and ensures that folic acid remains active in the digestive system. Take up to 500 mg daily.*

▶ *The vitamin B complex is also important. Vitamins B_6, B_{12}, and folic acid are all necessary for proper blood production and functioning.*

IRON-RICH DISHES FOR A VEGETARIAN

Because the iron in plant foods is less easily absorbed than the form found in animal foods, vegetarians must eat iron-rich plant foods at almost every meal to meet their daily needs. A sandwich of tempeh (a soy product) and watercress on whole-wheat bread accompanied by spinach is one good example of a meal that is high in iron. Bean soup with a whole-grain roll is another. (These also provide complete protein.)

Breakfast might include fortified cereal and soy milk. Dried fruits (especially apricots and prunes), peanuts, sunflower seeds, and roasted soybeans make excellent iron-rich snacks.

BOOSTING IRON
Spinach and other dark leafy greens; beans and other legumes; and whole-grain and enriched breads are very good sources of nonheme iron.

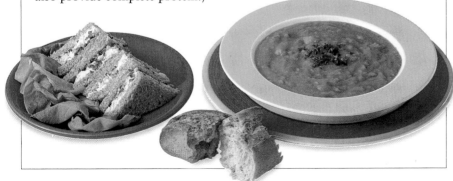

RESEARCH ON IRON DEFICIENCIES

A well-known study was conducted in the United States by Dr. Ernest Beutler in 1960. After giving 29 women who complained of fatigue a complete physical examination, he found that 22 had low iron stores and 7 had normal reserves. He gave them all placebo tablets for three months, followed by iron supplement tablets for three months. He then asked them which tablets had made them feel less fatigued. Although the response was mixed from the 7 normal women, out of the 22 who had low iron stores 15 said that the iron gave them more energy, 5 preferred the placebo, and 2 had no preference. Those who did not benefit from the supplements may have been unable to absorb the form of iron that the pills contained.

Adrenal Gland Problems

The adrenal glands provide hormones that are responsible for production of energy and many other bodily functions. Problems with these glands can lead to disorders that leave the body unable to cope with routine physical tasks.

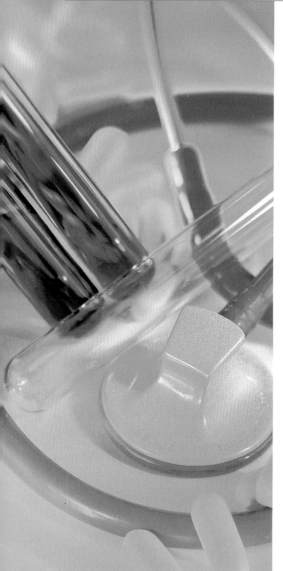

THE PROBLEMS

The adrenal glands, located on top of the kidneys, consist of two distinct parts that are responsible for producing very different hormones. The outer part, called the adrenal cortex, produces corticosteroid hormones and three hormones essential for reproduction—estrogen, progesterone, and androgen. The inner part, called the adrenal medulla, produces the hormones adrenaline and noradrenaline.

The corticosteroid hormones have a range of important effects on the body. One of them, aldosterone, helps to regulate fluid levels and so plays an important part in controlling blood pressure. Another one, hydrocortisone (or cortisol), controls the way the body uses certain nutrients, especially the breakdown of stored glucose during a crisis or period of extra physical exertion, and thus helps the body cope with stress. This hormone also affects the immune system and reduces inflammation. Androgens play an important part in female sex drive and a lesser part in male sex drive and sexual characteristics.

Adrenaline and noradrenaline are mainly released during times of stress. Their job is to prepare the body for activity by speeding up the heart and breathing rates and diverting blood to the muscles. When the body is exposed to long periods of stress, the adrenals can suffer.

ADRENAL GLAND FACTORS

Disorders of the adrenal glands can be prompted by a number of factors.

► *Infection*

► *Other glandular problems, particularly those involving the pituitary gland, which controls the adrenal gland to a great extent*

► *Addison's disease, a gradual failure of the adrenal glands*

► *Tumors, especially in major organs or glands, leading to an alteration of the hormonal system*

► *Prolonged stress or use of corticosteroids*

Because adrenal hormones have such varied effects, disorders of the glands can cause a wide range of symptoms. Signs of insufficient function include dehydration, with a consequent drop in blood pressure and risk of shock, hypoglycemia, weakness, dizziness, weight loss, and recurrent infections. Symptoms of excessive production include muscle wasting, weight gain and redistribution of fat to the trunk and upper back, menstrual problems, excessive facial hair, mental disorders, and mood swings. Production of some adrenal hormones is also influenced by the pituitary gland, and a tumor or other pituitary disorder can also lead to excess or reduced production of adrenal hormones.

SYMPTOMS

► Dehydration
► Drop in blood pressure
► Tiredness and fatigue
► Darkened skin
► Difficulty concentrating
► Dizziness
► Muscle wasting
► Unexplained weight gain or loss
► Recurrent infections

DIETARY MANAGEMENT

The adrenal glands depend not only on many nutrients for their optimum function but also on healthy activity on the part of the other glands in the endocrine system, such as the thyroid and pituitary. All these glands are strengthened by following a diet that provides an abundance of vegetables and fruits, complex carbohydrates (starches), and complete protein from sources such as meat, eggs, seafood, and soy products.

The adrenal glands require extra amounts of certain nutrients during periods of prolonged or intense stress because they tend to become depleted. Among them are vitamins B_5, B_6, and C, as well as magnesium and zinc, all of which are involved in the production of adrenal hormones. The B vitamins are plentiful in meat, whole grains, leafy vegetables, and legumes, which also contain zinc and magnesium. Peppers and citrus fruits are good sources of vitamin C.

The diet should also include foods to support the bacteria of the gut, which are responsible for producing such vitamins as pantothenic acid (B_5). Vegetable fiber provides a matrix for the acidophilus bacteria, which colonize the gut and may be replenished by bacteria-rich lacto-fermented foods, such as miso, tofu, and live yogurt, and by lacto-fermented juices. Celery juice is considered by some dietitians to be especially good for the adrenal glands.

Have regular meals that are high in complex carbohydrates and limit intake of sugar, tea, coffee, and alcohol to prevent fluctuations in blood sugar levels and minimize the stress on the adrenals. Snacking between meals can be a good way to balance your energy levels, as long as the snacks are healthful. Eat nuts, fruit, air-popped popcorn, or whole-grain crackers when you feel energy levels dropping a few hours after a meal.

SUPPLEMENTS

Supplements can help to ensure a proper intake of certain nutrients.

▶ *Several of the B vitamins, notably folic acid, B_5, and B_{12}, may protect against exhaustion.*

▶ *Vitamin C levels are significantly reduced under stressful conditions. Take 500 mg daily.*

▶ *Coenzyme Q10 as a supplement is thought to help ease various forms of fatigue and adrenal exhaustion, although there is no conclusive evidence. Take 30 mg daily.*

▶ *Magnesium plays an important role in regulating energy metabolism. Take 250 mg daily in the form of magnesium phosphate.*

▶ *Potassium is crucial for neuromuscular coordination, and additional quantities are needed in cases of fatigue. Use in a physiologically balanced formula combined with magnesium.*

HERBAL MEDICINE

A few herbs may support the adrenal glands by assisting the body's adaptation to stressful situations. Principal among these is ginseng *(Panax quinquefolius)*, which grows in shady woodlands of eastern and midwestern North America. It contains compounds known as adaptogens, which support the body's adaptive mechanisms to stressful situations and improve energy, alertness, and immune function as well. Ginseng may be taken for

GINSENG
Ginseng should be taken with care; too much can bring on an adrenaline rush or make it difficult to sleep at night.

three to four weeks at a time, followed by a break of two weeks before starting a course again. The usual dose is ½ to 1 teaspoon of extract in tea or juice, or the powdered root can be brewed as a tea.

Aromatherapy can also soothe stress. Lavender and the Bach Rescue Remedy are often advised for anxious situations.

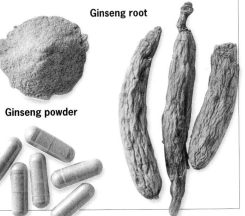

Ginseng root

Ginseng powder

Ginseng tablets

HOMEOPATHY

Homeopathy aims to cure an illness or condition through minute doses of plant extracts and other naturally occurring materials. The following remedies, which may help in the treatment of adrenal deficiency, should be taken in low potencies for a few weeks. Check your symptoms for the right remedy and see your doctor if symptoms persist.

Calcaria carbonicum 6 should be taken if you have a sallow complexion, cold extremities, nausea, low appetite, and insomnia. Natrum muriaticum 6 is for a yellow complexion, brown spots on the backs of the hands, lassitude, cold extremities, and tension in the kidney region. Sepia 6 should be taken for weakness, fainting, yellow complexion, nausea at the smell of food, weak back, and restless limbs.

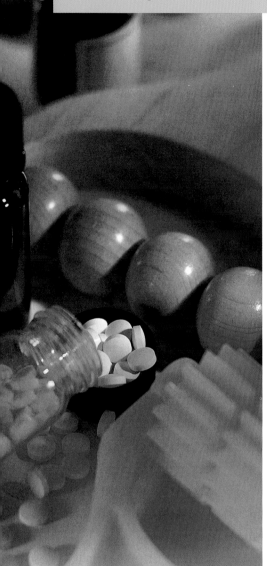

Thyroid Problems

The thyroid gland is in direct control of your metabolic rate and energy levels. Thyroid disorders are easily treated with orthodox medication, but alternative therapies and self-help measures can also help relieve symptoms and boost health.

THE PROBLEMS

The thyroid gland, situated at the front of the neck just below and in front of the voice box, produces two hormones—triiodothyronine (T3) and thyroxin (T4)—that regulate the rate at which cells convert food into energy. Both overproduction (hyperthyroidism) and underproduction (hypothyroidism) can have a serious effect on all bodily functions. Swelling of the thyroid gland (goitre) may occur with either condition, but it is more common in the latter.

To function properly, the thyroid needs iodine—found in seafood and plants grown in iodine-rich soil—and thyroid-stimulating hormone (TSH), produced by the pituitary gland. A deficiency or excess of either substance can lead to thyroid problems. Iodine deficiency is rare in North America, however, because of the availability of iodized salt.

Babies born with thyroid deficiency are at great risk for developing cretinism, a severe form of mental retardation and abnormal growth, unless treatment begins within the first few weeks of life. All babies born in hospitals in the United States are tested for thyroid deficiency.

Thyroid disorders can occur at any age, but because the symptoms are the same as those of many other conditions, they are often hard to detect. Medical intervention is essential, however. Your doctor can arrange for blood tests. A deficiency

of T4 accompanied by an increase of TSH indicates thyroid deficiency, for which the doctor may prescribe thyroxin tablets. If there are indications of an overactive thyroid, conventional treatment will be with drugs that suppress T4 or, in severe cases, surgical removal of part or all of the gland. When this is done, thyroxin tablets may have to be taken for life to counter the deficiency.

In borderline cases—such as those with normal test results but a persistence of symptoms—nutritional and/or herbal support may be effective (see opposite page).

THYROID FACTORS

Thyroid disorders can be triggered by female sex hormones or pregnancy (women with thyroid problems outnumber men five to one). They may also be a response to a severe infection, a pituitary tumor, excessive stress, or occupational hazards, especially exposure to radiation and certain industrial chemicals.

The thyroid can also be adversely affected by antibodies produced by the immune system (autoimmune disorder). With Hashimoto's disease, antibodies destroy the thyroid gland, resulting in hypothyroidism. In Grave's disease, antibodies stimulate the thyroid to produce excessive amounts of hormones, leading to hyperthyroidism.

SYMPTOMS

Of hypothyroidism
► Lethargy and lack of energy
► Unexplained weight gain
► Dry skin; thinning hair and nails
► Voice changes
► Sensitivity to cold

Of hyperthyroidism
► Palpitations and sweating
► Unexplained weight loss
► Protruding eyes
► Irritability and insomnia

DIETARY ADVICE

Dietary measures can be of help in avoiding a thyroid imbalance and for enhancing treatment of either hyperthyroidism or hypothyroidism.

The Iodine Factor

Both too much and too little iodine can cause the thyroid gland to malfunction. The daily need for iodine is no more than 150 mcg for adolescents and adults. Most people in North America easily meet this requirement, but exceptions may occur in Midwestern regions where the soil is poor in iodine. Natural sources of iodine include seafood and vegetables grown in iodine-rich soil. Iodized salt is a very good source, providing daily needs with just a little more than 1/2 teaspoon. Intake of iodine beyond 1,000 mcg per day is not advised.

Vitamins and minerals

Problems of insufficient thyroid hormones can be more severe when vitamin A is lacking at the same time. Fortified dairy products, liver, fish, yellow and orange vegetables and fruits, and dark leafy greens are good sources. However, the cruciferous vegetables—cabbage, cauliflower, and broccoli, for example—inhibit the effects of thyroid hormones when eaten raw. (This actually benefits people who produce excess thyroid.) Vitamins B_2, B_3, B_6, C, and E, and the mineral zinc are also involved in the manufacture of thyroid hormones. A deficiency may cause lower levels of them.

People with an overactive thyroid need additional calcium because they excrete it more quickly. They also need extra calories until their medication takes effect.

SUPPLEMENTS

Some nutritional supplements can improve thyroid problems. Consult a physician, howevver, before exceeding the daily recommendations.

► *Vitamin B complex provides metabolic support for cases of hyperthyroidism, but may also be a general tonic for the tiredness of hypothyroidism. Use 100 mg daily.*

► *Up to 400 mg per day of magnesium can help. Take as a combination with potassium.*

► *Vitamin E is a tonic to the circulation. Two capsules of 100 I.U. can be taken twice a day.*

► *Kelp, a preparation of the seaweed Fucus vesiculosus, is a source of natural iodine. Some health practitioners recommend kelp for thyroid problems; others advise against it because it can worsen them.*

STRESS MANAGEMENT

The pressures of long-term stress or anxiety can overexcite an already excessively active thyroid or place impossible demands on a deficient one. It is worth taking steps to lower your level of agitation and help the nervous system to function at a less demanding pace.

This can be achieved partly with a healthy diet that limits such stimulants as coffee, strong tea, and alcohol, and partly with exercise. Not only does exercise reduce stress, but it also stimulates the thyroid gland to secrete more hormones.

Practicing regular relaxation or meditation is very helpful. Yoga is an especially good technique because the gentle exercise and breathing routines are harmonizing to bodily functions (see page 116). Bach flower remedies may also be of help (see page 46). Aromatherapy massage using

essential oils is another method for managing stress. You can add several drops of oil to a warm bath or mix a few drops with a teaspoonful of water in an oil burner.

SELF-MASSAGE
The calming effects of massage with aromatherapy oils help to relieve stress.

HOMEOPATHY

Homeopathy is a gentle and safe way of supporting conventional treatment for thyroid problems, but you must follow the instructions carefully. For individualized deeper-acting prescriptions, you should consult a homeopath, but the following remedies may help in appropriate circumstances:

► *Fucus 6 can help to bring T4 down. Take one tablet four times daily.*

► *Spongia 30 increases T4 and is good for treating swollen glands and hard phlegm in the throat and voice changes. Take one tablet twice daily.*

► *Iodum 30 raises T4 and can slow an overactive thyroid and reduce restlessness. Take one tablet twice daily for two weeks.*

► *Belladonna 6 also raises T4 and helps hot, flushed hyperthyroid sufferers. Take one tablet four times daily for four or five days.*

Diabetes

Diabetes can come on gradually, rendering the sufferer progressively more tired and less able to transform food into energy. Dietary measures can help alleviate the problem and make it possible to resume a normal life.

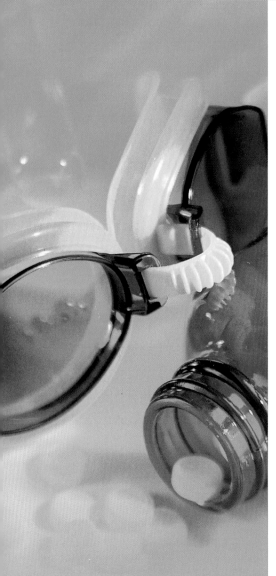

THE PROBLEM

Insulin, produced in the pancreas, promotes the uptake of glucose into cells so that it can be metabolized to produce energy. When the process is disturbed, either because of insufficient insulin or inability of the body to utilize it, blood sugar rises because it cannot get into the cells. The result is the disease known as diabetes.

There are two main types. The severest form—insulin-dependent (IDD), or type I, diabetes—most often occurs in young people. This needs to be treated with careful monitoring of blood sugar levels, insulin injections, and a strict diet.

The more common form—non-insulin-dependent (NIDD), or type II, diabetes—generally occurs later in life, usually after age 40, most often in overweight people. Because only about one-third of sufferers develop any symptoms, it may be discovered only as a result of routine medical tests, and thousands of people could be suffering from a mild form without realizing it. NIDD is often treated with dietary measures alone.

Diet is the most important factor in managing diabetes. After a meal the blood glucose level rises, and insulin is needed to transport it into body cells to be converted into energy. If the glucose cannot be transformed, the blood sugar rises to dangerous levels and the body cells are deprived of energy. Excess sugar is excreted in the urine and can be detected by tests.

CAUSES OF DIABETES

Insulin-dependent diabetes results from the destruction of insulin-secreting cells in the pancreas. It tends to run in families and is thought to be caused by the immune system attacking the body's own tissues, possibly following a viral infection. It occurs most often in people under the age of 16.

Non-insulin-dependent diabetes is caused by a reduction in the amount of insulin that is produced by the body or by the body becoming resistant to its effects. It is more common in overweight people who are middle-aged or older.

It is important that IDD diabetics follow a strict dietary regimen in order to balance carbohydrate consumption with insulin intake. The aim is to avoid sudden swings in blood sugar levels. This often requires discipline that can be hard to maintain, especially in children.

In particular, diabetics should limit their intake of simple sugars, which pass rapidly into the bloodstream and cause a sudden rise in blood glucose, and eat meals at regularly spaced times. Those taking insulin or tablets may also need snacks between meals and before bed. A dietitian can provide special guidelines on obtaining just the right amount of carbohydrate at each meal.

SYMPTOMS

► Tiredness and possibly dizziness and fainting
► Unusual thirst
► Excessive urination
► Unexplained weight loss
► Poor resistance to infections
► Tingling in the hands and feet
► Deterioration of eyesight

DIETARY MEASURES FOR DIABETICS

A number of dietary measures can help control blood glucose levels.

Carbohydrates

Simple sugars and foods that contain them, such as candies, cookies, and fruit drinks, should be consumed sparingly and, when possible, combined with a complex carbohydrate.

The main sources of energy should come from complex carbohydrates, such as bread, potatoes, millet, and rice. When these foods include the fiber (the bran of grains, the skin of potatoes), they are absorbed more slowly by the digestive system and thus keep blood sugar levels steadier.

Fruits and vegetables, excellent sources of fiber, are important also for their vitamins and minerals. Eat at least five portions every day.

Proteins

Protein from such plant sources as legumes, especially soybeans, provide additional fiber and can be included abundantly in the diet. Moderate quantities of animal protein from lean meats, fish, and low-fat dairy products are recommended.

Fats

Becauses fats can interfere with the action of insulin, they should be restricted to 15 to 20 percent of the diet and obtained mainly from plant sources, like seeds, nuts, and unsaturated vegetable oils.

HERBAL TREATMENT

A number of medicinal plants promote or support the functions of organs and tissues that are at risk from diabetes. The heart and circulatory system can be sustained with the help of hawthorn berries (*Crataegus oxyacantha*) and concentrated leaf extract of gingko biloba, reputed also to protect against diabetic retinopathy. Liver function can be aided by using barberry (*Berberis vulgaris*); the digestive system can be improved by using ginger (*Zingiber officinalis*); and immune function can be strengthened with garlic (*Allium sativum*).

DIABETIC HERBS
*There is evidence that fresh garlic cloves help control blood sugar, as well as to support the immune system. Some herbalists also recommend stinging nettle (*Urtica dioica*) tea, but this advice is not supported by medical doctors.*

Cinnamon has shown promise for use in Type II diabetes; $\frac{1}{8}$ to $\frac{1}{4}$ teaspoon of ground cinnamon taken at mealtimes may triple the body's insulin efficiency. Another herb recommended for use by diabetics is dandelion (in tea made with the roots and leaves).

SUPPLEMENTS

Research in nutritional biochemistry has revealed the importance of specific nutrients in stabilizing blood sugar levels, as well as helping to protect tissues susceptible to damage in diabetics. The heart, blood vessels, nervous system, and retinas in the eyes are particularly vulnerable, and antioxidant nutrients can help prevent their deterioration. It may be worth consulting a naturopath or a doctor who practices nutritional medicine for individual prescriptions and recommendations, especially if you are an insulin-dependent diabetic.

▶ *Chromium combines with other nutrients to form what is known as the glucose tolerance factor, which is particularly important for elderly diabetics. Glucose tolerance factor is found in brewer's yeast, and you may need to take up to 20 brewer's yeast tablets every day to satisfy your body's needs.*

▶ *Vitamin C is necessary for healthy tissues, especially those of the blood vessels, and to regulate cholesterol levels, which are inclined to be higher in diabetics. Take 500 to 1,000 mg daily, preferably in two doses, one with breakfast in the morning and the other with your evening meal, in the form of bioflavonoid complex.*

▶ *Multimineral supplements that contain the RDA or RNI of zinc, magnesium, and potassium—all of which are important in the regulation of blood sugar levels—should be taken daily. Health practitioners may also recommend additional supplements of individual minerals and trace elements.*

▶ *Evening primrose oil, which contains gamma linoleic acid (GLA) can help with metabolizing of essential fatty acids and boosting of energy levels. This is useful because many diabetics tend to be less efficient at this process.*

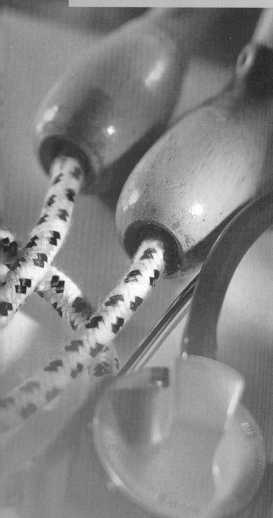

Hypoglycemia

Hypoglycemia, or low blood sugar, can cause tiredness and other more alarming symptoms. Dietary control to keep carbohydrate, protein, and fat intakes balanced is one of the primary methods of countering the condition.

THE PROBLEM

The body requires a steady supply of glucose, derived from food, for energy. But in order for glucose to be taken up by the cells, insulin, a hormone secreted by the pancreas, is needed. A lack of insulin causes hyperglycemia (excess sugar in the blood), which is a sign of diabetes (see page 142). If too much insulin is present, the blood glucose level falls too low, the condition known as hypoglycemia. This state is less critical for muscles and organs than it is for the brain because glucose is the only form of energy that the brain can use effectively. A severe case of hypoglycemia that goes uncorrected can progress to convulsions, coma, and even death.

Constant overproduction of insulin through excessive intake of sugary foods, a condition known as hyper-insulinism, can cause the body tissues to become gradually more resistant to insulin's influence. The wide range of symptoms thought to be due to insulin resistance have become known as syndrome X. They include chronic fatigue, allergies, headaches, loss of ability to concentrate, and irritability, as well as high blood pressure and cholesterol levels.

An accurate way of diagnosing hypoglycemia is with a glucose tolerance test, which measures the blood sugar levels at regular intervals for up to five hours after a concentrated glucose solution is taken. In a positive result, the blood sugar level actually falls below the fasting level after two-and-a-half to three hours and may be accompanied by headaches or a feeling of faintness. The rate at which the blood sugar level falls and the time it takes to recover give the technician important information about the type of hypoglycemia. It is also possible to diagnose hypoglycemia on the basis of clinical symptoms alone.

SYMPTOMS

Mild cases
▶ Inability to concentrate
▶ Frequent headaches
▶ Irritability and mood swings
▶ Persistent tiredness
▶ Frequent hunger pangs
▶ Depression

Severe cases
▶ Intense palpitations
▶ Cold and clammy skin or profuse sweating
▶ Blurred vision and dizziness
▶ Weakness and confusion

HYPOGLYCEMIA FACTORS

Most cases of hypoglycemia occur in people who have diabetes and who fail to eat regularly, take too much insulin or too high a dose of a hypoglycemic drug (prescribed for Type II diabetes), or exercise too strenuously. They experience a rapid fall of blood sugar levels, which produces some of the severe symptoms described in the far left column. The usual remedy is to take fruit juice or candy or, if unconscious, to be given injections of glucose or glucagon.

Hypoglycemia in nondiabetics can occur during a prolonged fast, as a side effect of certain medications, or when a tumor in the pancreas or pituitary gland alters insulin levels. The chances of developing hypoglycemia are greatly increased by over-consumption of caffeine, alcohol, and sugar, which produce a roller-coaster rise and fall of blood sugar.

DIETARY MANAGEMENT

A low-calorie diet made up mostly of carbohydrates can produce mild symptoms of hypoglycemia even if blood sugar levels remain in the low–normal range. The symptoms are temporarily alleviated by taking in more carbohydrates, but the cycle keeps repeating itself. The way to break the cycle is to eat regular meals that contain some protein and fat, because these take longer to digest and thus provide a steady release of energy, and to snack on foods that contain some fiber. Soluble fiber in particular—found in many fruits, nuts, seeds, and some vegetables—helps to control blood sugar levels.

Limit intake of refined foods

Avoid foods that release sugar too rapidly and overstimulate the pancreas. These include all refined carbohydrates, especially sugar and white flour. Also, limit intake of stimulants, particularly the caffeine in coffee, tea, and soft drinks. Too much alcohol can influence insulin production as well, and it interferes with the normal utilization of glucose.

Do not miss meals

Skipping any meal, but breakfast in particular, is sure to cause a drop in blood sugar. If regular mealtimes are difficult to achieve, keep on hand snacks such as yogurt, cheese and whole-grain crackers, and fruit.

Lifestyle and metabolism

Exercise regularly, building up the amount gradually. Also practice a relaxation routine and learn to take deep breaths. A tendency to hyperventilate (take rapid, shallow breaths) is common among people who are hypoglycemic.

SUPPLEMENTS

Nutritional supplements are no substitute for a healthy diet, but when used in conjunction with a balanced range of foods, they can help to prevent fluctuations in blood sugar levels. Vitamin B, magnesium, potassium, manganese, chromium, and zinc all play major roles in the regulation of blood sugar.

If you have pronounced symptoms of hypoglycemia, you should consult a doctor and have the appropriate tests. The tests commonly used for trace elements and minerals in blood serum are not as reliable indicators of their availability to the body as tests of the red blood cells.

The following supplements may be needed for hypoglycemia regulation and may be taken for three to six months at a time. Longer supplementation may be required by chronic sufferers of the syndrome.

▶ *Vitamin B complex at a dosage of 100 mg per day.*

▶ *Vitamin C, a 500 mg tablet taken twice daily.*

▶ *Magnesium doses of 200–400 mg per day, as magnesium orotate or physiologically balanced magnesium phosphate.*

▶ *Potassium, 500 mg per day, as a combination or as potassium phosphate, the physiologically balanced form.*

▶ *Zinc, 25 mg per day, taken at night before going to bed.*

▶ *Chromium, one of the most important nutrients in the control of blood sugar, combines with other compounds to form the glucose tolerance factor that is found in brewer's yeast. Brewer's yeast tablets supply the necessary factor. Preparations of chromium with magnesium and potassium can also be taken. The recommended dose is 200 mcg every day.*

ENERGY-BOOSTING SNACKS

Snacking between meals can help keep blood sugar levels steady. While it is often easier to reach for a candy bar or some cookies, the refined sugar and flour in such foods raise blood sugar levels too rapidly, and they will drop just as quickly. Snacks that contain fiber are digested more slowly, providing a constant stream of fuel to carry you through to the next meal. Good high-energy snacks include fresh and dried fruits; nuts and seeds, especially raw ones; raw vegetables, like carrots, sweet peppers, cauliflower, snow peas, and celery, either on their own or with low-fat dips; rice cakes, whole-grain crackers, or bread; low-calorie whole-grain breakfast cereals; low-fat and nonfat yogurts; air-popped popcorn; cheese such as Cheddar and low-fat cottage cheese.

ENERGY FOODS
You can eat as many pieces of fresh fruit and vegetables as you like to keep your energy levels high.

Cancer

Cancer is the cause of one out of every four deaths in North America, and it can affect people of all ages, although it is more common in older age groups. Understanding the many possible causes of cancer can help you take steps to avoid it.

THE PROBLEM

Cancer is an uncontrolled malignant growth of cells in any part of the body, though it most often affects the lungs, breasts, skin, reproductive organs, stomach, large bowel, pancreas, and the blood and bone marrow. A cancerous tumor grows and spreads into surrounding tissues, where it destroys nerves and erodes bones. It may also travel (metastasize) to other parts of the body through the blood vessels or lymphatic system, creating satellite tumors.

The hallmark of a cancerous, or malignant, tumor is that it spreads. A tumor that does not spread is said to be "benign" and is considered less dangerous, although it may still be life-threatening if it presses on a vital organ, such as the brain.

Symptoms of cancer vary enormously according to the site of the tumor. General fatigue and unexplained weight loss are common symptoms of the early stages of many cancers. Pain is not often an early symptom, although it should always be investigated by your doctor.

The main trigger factors are alcohol, smoking, ultraviolet light from the sun, diets, especially those high in animal fats or smoked foods, and environmental pollutants that are breathed in or consumed in food and drinking water. Some people are at particular risk for genetic reasons.

Many cancers that occur in adulthood are also related to changes in the cells due to aging. People under 20 years old are the least likely to contract cancer; the probability doubles after 30 and increases steadily throughout life. By the time a person reaches 90, there is a strong likelihood that he or she will have developed some form of cancer, although it may remain dormant and without symptoms.

Cancer is now the most common cause of death in North America, accounting for 27 percent, or roughly one in four, of all deaths. It has been identified since ancient times and also occurs in the animal kingdom.

Orthodox treatment for cancer includes one or more of the following: powerful drugs (chemotherapy), radiation (radiotherapy), and surgery. Many people use alternative health therapies in addition to help boost the immune system and alleviate some symptoms of cancer, as well as the side effects of treatment.

Some of the most effective complementary therapies are homeopathic and herbal treatments. A healthy and nutritious diet that includes plenty of the antioxidant vitamins found in fresh fruits and vegetables and whole-grain cereals will also strengthen the body. Visualization and art therapy, designed to focus the individual's own mental and physical resources on destroying the cancer, have also shown remarkable results.

SYMPTOMS

Cancer can have a wide range of possible symptoms, including

▶ Fatigue and rapid weight loss

▶ A persistent sore or ulcer

▶ A mole that changes size

▶ Severe headaches or persistent abdominal pain

▶ Blood in the urine

▶ Changes to, or unexplained lumps in, the breasts or testicles

▶ Abnormal vaginal bleeding

FACTORS INFLUENCING THE RISK OF CANCER

Food and diet
Up to 70 percent of cancers are thought to be linked to diet, especially one that is high in animal fats and refined sugar. Stomach cancer is highest in countries like Japan, where a lot of smoked foods are eaten. Bowel cancer is most common in countries where diets are low in fiber, such as Canada and the United States.

Environment
The most common environmental cause of cancer is ultraviolet light from the sun. This can cause such skin cancers as malignant melanoma. Less common factors include asbestos and radioactivity—both natural and man-made.

Genetic
Certain genes, passed on from one generation to the next, make it more likely that particular tisues, especially in the female reproductive organs, may turn cancerous. So far only a few "cancer genes" have been found, representing a minority of cancers.

Smoking and alcohol
Smoking is by far the most common cause of lung cancer. Excess alcohol consumption increases the risk of developing cancers of the esophagus (gullet), stomach, and liver.

Viruses
The human papillomavirus, which causes genital warts, has been strongly linked to cervical cancer, and the hepatitis B virus can cause liver cancer. Infection by the human immunodeficiency virus (HIV) increases the risk of developing a range of cancers. These viruses are most commonly contracted through unprotected sexual intercourse. Other viruses may also cause cancer, but in many cases the link is not clear.

A HEALTHY DIET
The main secret of a healthy diet is balance and moderation. Avoid excessive consumption of high-fat animal foods, refined sugars, and smoked meat, fish, and cheese. Also avoid highly processed foods and those with large quantities of additives. Eat plenty of different kinds of fruits and vegetables to ensure the maximum intake of antioxidants and other phytonutrients that help prevent cancer. Eat plenty of high-fiber foods, such as legumes and whole-grain cereals. Fiber speeds waste products through the digestive tract and reduces the time that cancer-causing substances are in contact with the body. A diet that is high in soy products, such as soybeans and tofu, is thought to reduce the risk of breast cancer.

PREVENTION OF SKIN CANCER

Skin cancer affects an increasing number of people every year, especially those with fair skin who have not protected themselves against the harmful ultraviolet rays of the sun. Staying out of the sun, wearing protective clothing, and using cream with a sun protective factor of 30 can reduce the risk of skin cancer. Pigmentations that are potentially cancerous should be examined yearly.

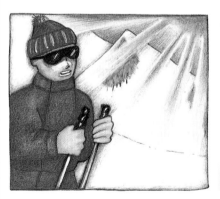

A holiday in the snow can increase the risk of skin cancer dramatically. This is because snow reflects the sun's rays, increasing the amount of ultraviolet rays received.

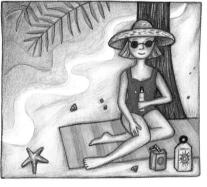

A holiday in the sun can be highly dangerous for fair-skinned people, particularly those with very pale skin that burns easily. Everyone should sunbathe carefully and with good protection.

LIFESTYLE FACTORS
The best way to reduce the risk of contracting cancer is to follow a healthy lifestyle. This means making sure that the body is as fit as possible and also avoiding those factors known to increase the risk of cancer, including excessive alcohol consumption, smoking, unprotected sunbathing, and a diet high in fat and low in fiber. Regular moderate exercise, such as brisk walking, golf, swimming, or cycling, will strengthen the body's immune system. Exercise should not, however, become excessive, which can have the opposite effect on health.

Women should examine their breasts regularly, and men should examine their testicles to check for lumps or other abnormalities. Women should also have regular PAP smear tests and mammograms.

HIV and AIDS

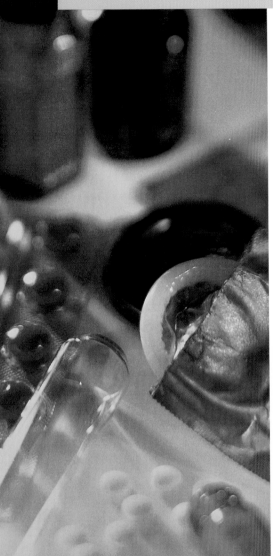

AIDS is an incurable disorder, caused by the HIV virus, that is spreading rapidly in countries around the world. The only way to avoid contracting the infection is to take proper precautions in intimate situations.

THE PROBLEM

AIDS stands for acquired immune deficiency syndrome. As the word syndrome indicates, the condition covers a wide range of possible disorders that may develop following the breakdown of the immune system. AIDS is caused by infection with the human immunodeficiency virus (HIV), which is most commonly contracted through infected blood, semen, or vaginal secretions. The infection may also be passed from mother to baby during childbirth or breastfeeding, although this can now be prevented. In the past HIV was also acquired from infected blood and blood products used during medical procedures. This is no longer a risk in most countries because blood donors are screened and blood products are heat-treated to kill the virus.

AIDS first came to the attention of doctors in 1981, when a rare lung infection affecting previously healthy homosexual men in the United States was reported. A series of infections, mostly rare in people who have properly functioning immune systems, spread throughout this community and were also discovered in intravenous drug users and hemophiliacs, which suggested that infection was through the blood. In 1984 American and French researchers identified the HIV virus.

HIV targets the T4 white cells in the bloodstream, which are a vital line of defense against disease. The immune system becomes seriously weakened, leaving the sufferer highly vulnerable to a range of opportunistic infections and cancers that a healthy person would probably fight off. HIV may also damage the brain and nervous system directly.

The interval between contracting HIV and developing the syndrome in its most serious form, known as "full-blown AIDS," can be months or even years. Some people develop a milder condition called AIDS-related complex (ARC), in which they may have periods of good health interspersed with periods of illness. While many people with HIV infection do not show symptoms, they are still infectious. The spread of the disease can be stopped only by following certain precautions, which can easily be understood and adopted.

CAUSES OF INFECTION

The virus can be passed from person to person in a variety of ways, all of which can be avoided.

► *Unprotected sexual intercourse with an infected person*

► *Blood transfusion with infected blood (now very rare)*

► *Through the uterus, blood, or breast milk of an infected mother*

► *The use of contaminated intravenous needles*

SYMPTOMS

Common minor symptoms include

► Skin disorders

► Unexplained weight loss

► Chronic diarrhea

► Fever

Severe symptoms include susceptibility to infections, such as

► Herpes

► Hepatitis

► Tuberculosis

► Cancerous tumors

DIAGNOSING AND TREATING HIV AND AIDS

HIV infection is diagnosed by means of a blood test to detect antibodies that the body produces to fight the disease. Those with HIV antibodies are said to be HIV positive. There is no cure as yet; HIV-positive people are infected for life and will always be able to pass on the virus. The test may yield a false negative if it is done within two to three months of infection, before the antibodies have had a chance to develop, or late in the disease, when the immune system has broken down completely.

Current orthodox treatments for HIV infection and AIDS are extending the life of sufferers by several years, and new treatments are being discovered all the time that further improve the outlook for patients.

Alternative health measures can also provide useful additional care. In particular they can help strengthen the immune system and alleviate some symptoms. They include homeopathic, herbal, and traditional Chinese therapies, which are most effective when supervised by qualified practitioners who specialize in AIDS.

In addition, people with HIV/AIDS can strengthen their immune system and help prevent or delay weight loss and other complications by following a healthy lifestyle that includes regular moderate exercise and management of stress levels. A well-balanced diet, one low in animal fats, sugar, and refined foods and high in whole-grain cereals, legumes, fruits, and vegetables, is also beneficial.

Because people with HIV are more vulnerable to infections, including food poisoning, they should pay special attention to food safety. Eat only well-done eggs, seafood, meat, and poultry. Wash all vegetables and fruits thoroughly, preferably eating them peeled and cooked or juiced.

HAVING A TEST

Should I have an HIV test?
It is very important to have a test for HIV if you think there is a chance you may have become infected or you are in a high-risk group, which includes people who have had unprotected sex with someone whose sexual history is unknown to them (kissing is not a risk). If you plan to have a test, seek counseling first for help in comprehending the implications of a positive test result.

Where do I get an HIV test?
Your own doctor can carry out a blood test for HIV, but if you prefer, tests for HIV are available at clinics that specialize in genitourinary disorders. The result is totally confidential, and the doctor or the clinic staff can give you counseling as well as medical advice and treatment.

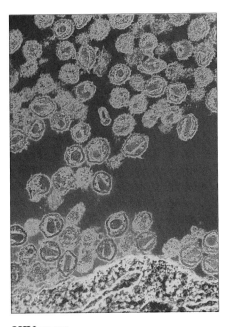

HIV VIRUS
The HIV virus affects the white blood cells, gradually crippling the immune system and leaving weak points that allow infections to take hold. Common infections that can easily breach a weakened immune system include herpes, pneumonia, hepatitis, and tuberculosis.

NUTRITIONAL SUPPLEMENTS AND HERBS

Many studies have shown that HIV-positive and AIDS patients tend to be deficient in certain nutrients because they absorb them poorly, suffer chronic diarrhea that depletes them, or are not consuming enough food as a result of poor appetite. Supplementation can play an important role in supporting the immune system and helping to slow the progression from HIV infection to full-blown AIDS. However, taking supplements should always be supervised by a dietitian or naturopath because large doses of some nutrients can be toxic or may worsen conditions they would normally help prevent. Very high doses of vitamin C, for example, can worsen diarrhea. Supplying optimum amounts of each nutrient is the goal, and new approaches are discovered every da..

A number of studies have indicated that antioxidants, including vitamins A, C, and E and the mineral selenium, as well as vitamin B_{12} (necessary for production of red blood cells), slow the progression of AIDS. In the case of vitamin A, its precursor, beta carotene, appears to be more effective (and less toxic) than the vitamin itself.

Zinc and vitamin B_6, always important for proper immune function, are often deficient in AIDS patients. Supplementation of these nutrients can be beneficial when given in the correct dosage.

A few herbs have shown promise in the treatment of HIV. Curcumin, the yellow pigment in turmeric (a key spice in curries), is one of them. It has anti-inflammatory and antioxidant properties, which may slow replication of the virus, and is soothing to the digestion and restorative to the liver. Another is licorice, which in several studies has improved the immune function of HIV patients without the side effects exhibited by conventional drugs.

Chronic Fatigue Syndrome, or ME

A complex array of symptoms makes chronic fatigue syndrome, also known as myalgic encephalomyelitis, an enigma to many people, but a number of measures can help to alleviate the condition and aid recovery.

THE PROBLEM

Chronic fatigue syndrome (CFS), or myalgic encephalomyelitis (ME), is a complex illness, a major feature of which is persistent, debilitating fatigue that lasts for at least six months. The onset of its symptoms, which are generally flulike, often follows a viral illness, so another name in common use is postviral fatigue syndrome. In the United States the disorder is sometimes referred to by the more comprehensive term *chronic fatigue immune deficiency syndrome (CFIDS)*.

The collection of names emphasizes how imprecise a condition it is. The symptoms affect the whole body, yet a complete physical examination, blood analyses, and other tests will usually show everything to be normal. Because no single pathological cause has been found to account for it, chronic fatigue syndrome remains a controversial illness.

At least two-thirds of sufferers are white middle-class women; many are depressed, so the disorder is often labeled as psychosomatic. The depression, however, is often an extension of the fatigue and not the underlying cause. Under investigation as possible causes are hormone deficiencies, allergies, neurological damage sustained in a previous illness, and reactivation of a dormant virus, such as the Epstein-Barr virus, which remains in the body for the lifetime of its host (see page 153).

CAUSES OF CFS (ME)

There is no single cause of CFS, but a number of factors that undermine immunity and energy metabolism may combine to precipitate the illness. They include the following.

► *Recurring viral illnesses*
► *Chronic insufficient sleep*
► *Poor nutrition*
► *Weaknesses in the digestive function*
► *Hypoglycemia*
► *Intestinal candidiasis (yeast overgrowth)*
► *Impaired liver function*
► *A prolonged period of intense stress*

Just as diagnosis of the disorder is controversial, so, too, is its treatment. So far, there is no single satisfactory solution to the problem, although commonsense regimens seem to be helpful. Good nutrition (perhaps enhanced with supplements), plenty of rest, and moderate exercise are among the more successful ways of dealing with CFS and some of the effects associated with its fatigue. Herbal and homeopathic remedies can also help moderate some of the symptoms. Relaxation practices have played a significant role in aiding recuperation in some cases. Recovery can take up to a year or two.

SYMPTOMS

CFS exhibits a combination of baffling symptoms.

► Extreme tiredness and inability to concentrate
► Joint aches and stiffness
► Mild fever
► Recurring headaches
► Recurring sore throats
► Insomnia or sleep that does not refresh
► Muscle weakness and pain
► Painful lymph nodes
► Sensitivity to bright light
► Short-term memory problems

MANAGEMENT OF CHRONIC FATIGUE SYNDROME

Sufferers of chronic fatigue syndrome should always seek professional advice. Because the condition is a collection of symptoms, there is no definitive test for it, but a number of disorders that have similar symptoms must be systematically ruled out. Among the conditions doctors look for are adrenal insufficiency, lupus, hypoglycemia, hypothyroidism, disorders of liver function, leukemia and other cancers, deficiencies of digestive enzymes or vitamins and minerals, and intestinal candidiasis. Certain medicinal drugs also produce fatigue as a side effect.

Chronic fatigue is the consequence of a number of possible ways in which energy production and nerve function have become obstructed or impaired by a viral infection or damage to the immune system. The sequence of physiological and biochemical reactions requires specific nutrients at various stages.

Nutrition

Dietary measures and nutritional supplements are important components of CFS management. A person with the disorder needs a diet that meets a number of criteria. However, a balanced food intake is of little value if the ability to digest or absorb food is impaired; the nutrients from food and supplements will not be assimilated. It is advisable to consult a clinical dietitian or naturopath, who can give advice on suitable dietary measures and supplements to meet your individual needs.

Ample amounts of whole-grain starches are required for energy, and lean meat, legumes, and other low-fat, high-protein foods are essential to build and maintain muscles. At least three or four servings of fruit and four of vegetables every day will provide the vitamins and minerals needed to resist infection (see box, right, for more dietary tips).

Alcohol, which lowers immunity, should be avoided, and caffeinated drinks should be kept to a minimum because they can exacerbate sleep problems, as well as cause blood sugar levels to fluctuate wildly.

Low blood pressure may contribute to the fatigue of some CFS patients. Such people may be salt resistant and will feel better with a higher salt intake through such foods as pickles, olives, and canned soups.

Exercise

Excessive aerobic exercise may worsen the condition of the CFS patient. Dr Paul Cheney, a leading authority in the United States, says patients with this disease cannot be trained aerobically unless they are well on the way to recovery. Aerobic exercise, like running, swimming, and cycling, must therefore be strictly rationed. Some studies suggest that graded daily exercise, such as walking or gentle swimming, building up the amount by small weekly increments, can help. Anaerobic exercise, such as weightlifting, seems to be more manageable for short periods.

NONSTRENUOUS EXERCISE
Singing is great for the lungs and improves heartbeat, blood oxygen levels, and a sense of well-being without bringing on exhaustion. Joining a community chorus or church choir can be good exercise for your cardiovascular system and an excellent way to reduce stress as well. If you find it too tiring to sing standing up, you can always sit down, provided you keep your back straight.

DIETARY TIPS

The following dietary tips have proved beneficial in many cases of CFS. However, always consult your doctor or a qualified nutritionist or naturopath before making major changes in your diet.

▶ *Consume unrefined complex carbohydrates, such as whole-wheat bread and cereals, brown rice, millet, bulgur, and quinoa.*

▶ *Have a mixed salad of raw fruits and vegetables every day.*

▶ *Eat at least seven servings of fruits and vegetables every day.*

▶ *Vary your protein intake with more legumes, nuts, seeds, and tofu in place of meat, eggs, and cheese. If you are not a vegetarian, oily fish once a week is recommended for its omega-3 fatty acids.*

▶ *Eat smaller, more frequent meals rather than three larger ones. Carry some sunflower or pumpkin seeds, nuts, or fruit for a snack in case you have to delay a meal.*

▶ *Avoid caffeine and alcohol, which overactivate the first phase of liver detoxification, producing more potent toxic compounds.*

▶ *Avoid sugar and foods that contain it, such as cake, cookies, and candy, which are a potential challenge to the digestive system as well as the metabolism.*

A MENU FOR CFS

This menu planner will give you some idea of the variety of foods that provide essential nutrients without placing stress on the liver, pancreas, and intestines. If you think you might have an allergy or intolerance to a particular type of food, make a note of how you feel when you have eaten it; should you notice any ill effects, cut it out of your diet and substitute another food that meets the same nutritional needs. By monitoring the effects of different foods, you can include only those that are best for you.

On rising

▶ A cup of hot water with a teaspoonful of apple cider vinegar or fresh lemon juice and half a teaspoon of honey stirred in; or one cup of pepper-mint tea.

Breakfast

▶ Fresh fruit juice

▶ Homemade muesli, made by soaking organic oats in a cup of water overnight and adding grated apple, sliced pear, or raisins, and pumpkin or sunflower seeds. Commercially made muesli is also appropriate but may be high in sugar.

▶ Yogurt with live cultures

▶ An herbal tea, such as peppermint or lemon-ginger, or decaffeinated tea or coffee

Midmorning

▶ Cup of peppermint, chamomile, rose hip, or other herbal tea

▶ A double handful of sunflower seeds, a few brazil nuts or almonds, or peanut butter on toast

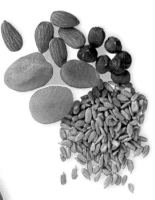

Lunch

▶ A mixed raw salad containing a selection of lettuce, watercress, parsley, white cabbage, chicory, cucumber, tomatoes, and carrots. Add a spoonful of part-skim ricotta or cottage cheese. Garnish with pine nuts, raisins, or pumpkin seeds and add a dressing of extra virgin olive oil, vinegar, and tahini or yogurt.

▶ Whole-grain crackers or bread or a baked potato with low-fat spread or hummus

▶ Fresh fruit for dessert

Dinner

▶ Aperitif of lacto-fermented beet or celery juice or a mixed vegetable juice

▶ A raw food appetizer of grated apple and carrot dressed with virgin olive oil and lemon juice; or crudités of carrot, pepper, celery, cauliflower, or broccoli and a tofu, hummus, or yogurt dip

▶ Main dish of fish, lean meat, or a vegetarian option served with two or three steamed vegetables; or vegetable stew made with fresh ingredients; or a brown rice or pasta dish. Do not fry the ingredients.

▶ Fresh fruit, a soy-based or yogurt-based dessert, soaked dried fruit, or a fruit sorbet or sherbet

Midafternoon

▶ A cup of herbal tea or a glass of fresh fruit juice.

▶ Seeds, nuts, or whole-grain crackers

▶ A piece of fresh fruit or a bowl of cut up fresh fruit

HERBAL TREATMENTS

A medical herbalist can select combinations of plant extracts according to the specific needs of the patient. Detoxification functions may be assisted by the use of barberry (*Berberis vulgaris*), pokeroot (*Phytolacca decandra*), especially for fatigue following mononucleosis, and burdock (*Arctium lappa*). Barberry is also an organ remedy for the liver, while pokeroot helps improve lymphatic functions.

Irritated or weakened intestinal linings may impair absorption of nutrients and cause food intolerances. They can be assisted by extracts of licorice (*Glycyrrhiza glabra*), which also supports the adrenal glands, marsh mallow (*Althea officinalis*), and wild yam (*Dioscoroea villosa*). Among general tonics are kola (*Cola vera*), especially for muscle weakness, damiana (*Turnera diffusa*), also a useful aphrodisiac, and wild oats (*Avena sativa*). Ginger (*Zingiber officinalis*) may be used to assist the actions of the other herbs and is a good digestive tonic.

There are a few herbs that may be tried without professional guidance, including ginseng (*Panax ginseng*), gingko (*Gingko biloba*), which helps improve circulation to the extremities, and coneflower (*Echinacea angustifolia*), which stimulates nonspecific immunity. Any of these may be taken for two to three weeks at a time, followed by a break of two to three weeks.

INFECTIOUS MONONUCLEOSIS

Mononucleosis is a highly contagious disease that strikes mostly adolescents and young adults. The Epstein-Barr virus (EBV), which causes the disease, has infected most children by age five, but the majority simply develop immunity and do not get sick. When symptoms do occur, they begin 30 to 60 days after exposure and include severe fatigue, as well as fever, sore throat, swollen lymph nodes, headache, and muscular pains. Symptoms usually persist for one to four weeks, but full recovery may take a few months.

Orthodox treatment involves regular rest and plenty of liquids, as well as careful monitoring to deal with any complications that may develop. Because the Epstein-Barr virus stays in the body throughout life, some health practitioners believe that it is implicated in chronic fatigue syndrome, though this has never been proved.

Dietary measures

Foods rich in vitamins and minerals that help to boost the immune system will hasten recovery. Important vitamins include A, plentiful in liver, eggs, fish oils, and low-fat dairy products; C, found in many fruits and vegetables; E, found in wheat germ, nuts, seeds, and vegetable oils; and the B complex, available in lean meat, fish, soybeans, peanuts, and other legumes, and whole-grain products. Significant minerals include copper, iron, selenium, and zinc, found in lean meat, fish, whole grains, and brown rice.

Some people may benefit from supplements, but this should be done with professional advice to avoid overdoses. It is always better to obtain the nutrients you need naturally from a well-balanced diet.

Homeopathy

A qualified homeopath tailors a remedy to an individual situation. However, the following have proved effective in many cases: Ailanthus for rash and inflammation; Mercurious solubilis for swollen lymph nodes and fatigue; Phytolacca for general aches and pains.

SUPPLEMENTS

You should seek a nutritionist's advice about which supplements would meet your specific needs and help improve both your energy levels and any underlying condition. However, the following supplements will invariably be helpful in most cases of chronic fatigue.

▶ *Vitamin B complex, a yeast-free type, at a dose of 100 mg per day.*

▶ *Vitamin C taken at 500–1000 mg per day divided in three doses.*

▶ *Vitamin E as two capsules of an emulsified form of the 100-mg strength, taken twice daily.*

▶ *Magnesium is one of the most important nutrients for chronic fatigue. This should be taken as magnesium citrate, 200 mg daily, or, in the physiologically balanced form, magnesium phosphate, combined with potassium phosphate, another nutrient important to combating fatigue.*

▶ *Zinc may be taken as zinc citrate 50 mg, two tablets daily. Take zinc supplements at night, separately from other nutrients.*

▶ *Selenium is found in brewer's yeast, together with the glucose tolerance factor, chromium. Use brewer's yeast tablets if you do not have yeast-related digestive problems (candidiasis;, otherwise, use the commercially available combination of selenium with vitamins A and C. Selenium works closely with vitamin E, with which it should always be taken.*

▶ *Coenzyme Q10 might be beneficial, although there is no conclusive evidence to support this theory. However, it may be helpful as a supplement in cases that have muscle fatigue as a prominent feature. The recommended dose is 20–50 mg per day.*

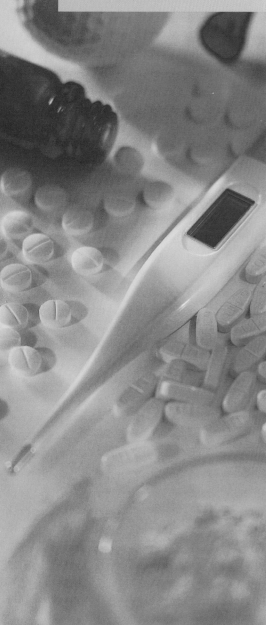

Viral Infections

Viral infections, which are often debilitating, can be alleviated by a number of alternative therapies, home remedies, and dietary regimens. Keeping your immune system in good health is the best way to prevent viruses from taking hold.

THE PROBLEM

Viruses are microorganisms that cause a wide range of diseases, from colds and influenza to AIDS and some forms of cancer. Chickenpox, cold sores, shingles, and glandular fever are all viral illnesses.

Containing a core of nucleic acid surrounded by protein, viruses invade weakened cells of the body and multiply within them, eventually causing their death. When this happens on a large enough scale, vast areas of tissue may be severely damaged or even destroyed. Local or general symptoms of inflammation or fever may occur, indicating that the body's immune system is at work and its defensive cells are attempting to destroy invading viruses.

Once the immune system recognizes a virus as being harmful, it can produce antibodies against future invaders of the same type of virus. However, many viruses are capable of transforming themselves into strains that the immune system does not recognize or more virulent ones that may cause more severe health problems than the original version.

Many viral illnesses are debilitating, placing great demands on the body's energy reserves. The increased burden of detoxification placed on the liver and organs of elimination may leave feelings of sluggishness and lethargy, which are often made worse by the treatments commonly used to relieve infections.

SYMPTOMS

► Fever
► Inflammation in specific areas of the body
► Fatigue, lethargy, and constant tiredness
► Pain and aching muscles
► Swollen glands

IMMUNE HEALTH FACTORS

Certain factors have a detrimental effect on the immune system.

► *Alcohol depresses levels of vitamin B and zinc, which are essential to immune competence. It can also reduce the uptake of several other crucial nutrients.*

► *Cigarette smoking actually raises the white blood cell count, activating the immune system. However, smoking also causes low-grade chronic bronchitis.*

► *Toxic points—areas of localized infection, such as dental abscesses or infected tonsils—may disturb the normal processes of neutralization and elimination and weaken the cellular defenses.*

► *The repeated use of drugs, such as corticosteroids and broad-spectrum antibiotics, to treat infections, destroys beneficial acidophilus bacteria in the gut, which play an important defensive role.*

► *Deficiencies of many nutrients, especially certain vitamins, and minerals, have been associated with depression of the immune system.*

► *Prolonged stress reduces the effectiveness of the immune system and is often a contributing factor to a weakened immune response.*

► *Excessive exercise may depress the immune system temporarily.*

► *Lack of natural daylight is associated with a greater level of illness and infection.*

IMMUNE SYSTEM FUNCTIONING

Our bodies have a sophisticated defense system that consists of specialized cells found in the lymph glands, spleen, bone marrow, intestines, and lungs. These tissues produce white blood cells, which either engulf invading viruses or bacteria or produce antibodies that neutralize foreign cells. The sinuses, lungs, and intestines are lined with immunoglobulins, and blood levels of these substances can be measured to assess immune activity.

We are born with passive immunity, a basic system of defense cells ready to deal with invaders of almost any sort. This nonspecific immunity is reinforced through the breast milk. Further immunity is acquired through the formation of antibodies during viral attacks, for example, such childhood illnesses as measles and chickenpox.

Why do viral illnesses occur?

Many factors can undermine our immunity. In the past, poor standards of hygiene and inadequate nutrition were held responsible for major epidemics, and to a great extent this is still true in many underdeveloped areas of the world.

Now, however, diseases of excess are more prevalent in the developed world. Excesses of food processing, chemical residues in food, and even hygiene—as represented by a preoccupation with combating illness through the overprescription of antibiotics—have all contributed to a gradual erosion of immune competence. In addition, other aspects of modern life, such as air conditioning, central heating, electromagnetic radiation, and atmospheric pollution, have been implicated in the growing susceptibility to viral illnesses.

Preventing viral infections

Although there are many factors that increase susceptibility to infections, and avoiding them will undoubtedly help, there are also a number of measures that can sustain and strengthen immune response, among them, herbalism and naturopathy.

HERBAL REMEDIES

An herbalist may advise some herbs to support vulnerable organs and others to stimulate immunity.

▶ *Coneflower (Echinacea angustifolia) stimulates nonspecific resistance. Take capsules or 10–20 drops of tincture dissolved in hot water three times a day for up to two weeks.*

▶ *Ginseng (Panax ginseng) contains adaptogens, which help the body adjust to infections and stress. It is usually available as the crude herb root (you can steep a slice in hot water to use daily as a tea) or tablets of varying strength (use maximum recommended by the manufacturer).*

▶ *Licorice (Glycyrrhiza glabra) is an adrenal tonic that stimulates the formation of white blood cells and antibodies.*

▶ *Garlic (Allium sativum) is an antiseptic and blood cleanser, good for catarrhal infections. For best results, use raw garlic or tablets prepared from freeze-dried garlic.*

SELF-HELP FOR IMMUNE SUPPORT

A number of general measures can help stimulate your resistance to viral infections or to aid in your recovery when they are difficult to shake off. Many are based simply on common sense and the underlying principles of good health—exercise, relaxation, and a well-balanced, nutritious diet.

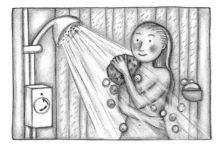

HYDROTHERAPY
Regular cold showers have a protective effect. A study comparing university students who had a daily cold shower with those who did not showed that those who took the cold showers had significantly fewer colds.

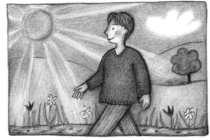

LIGHT
Evidence that people working under artificial light suffer from more infections than those exposed to natural light points to the positive effects of sunlight on health. It is well known that sunlight is essential for the formation of vitamin D.

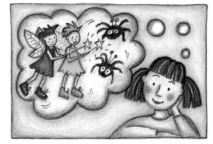

VISUALIZATION
In guided imagery a person focuses thoughts on the body's defenses, using images appropriate to his or her interests. For example, a child might imagine a team of fairies chasing a virus out of the blood.

DIETARY ADVICE

If you are prone to recurrent viral infections, the first recommendation is to review your eating habits. Avoid those foods and beverages that are proven suppressors of immunity and have regular meals with plenty of fresh vegetables and fruits and whole-grain products. Particular foods may have to be increased or reduced for specific types of viral infection. On example is herpes, for which foods containing the amino acid arginine (contained in nuts and seeds) need to be reduced and those containing the amino acid lysine (found in yogurt and cottage cheese) need to be increased.

There are also many foods that should feature regularly in your diet for their immune-sustaining and potentiating effects. Garlic and onions have antibacterial and antifungal properties. They also contain sulfur compounds that support detoxification functions of the liver. Yogurt with live cultures contains lactic acid bacteria, which have immune supportive properties. Lacto-fermented vegetable juices also provide lactic acid bacteria.

Vegetables and fruits are rich in the antioxidant vitamins C and A, which protect cells against damage from oxidation. The antioxidant vitamin E, plentiful in nuts, seeds, and leafy vegetables does the same. Poultry, seafood, Brazil nuts, legumes, and whole grains provide selenium, a trace element important for immune support and proper functioning. Zinc, found in shellfish, meat, poultry, eggs, legumes, yogurt, and whole grains also bolsters the immune system.

An important way of improving resistance to infections is through dietary modification, together with other measures like hydrotherapy, nutritional supplements, and herbal medicines. For the most appropriate way of integrating these for your personal requirements, consult a naturopath or dietitian.

SUPPLEMENTS

Keeping your body healthy and working to its best potential is an important aspect of immune protection against viral diseases, and a wide range of vitamins, minerals and trace elements play important roles in immune protection. Care should be taken to avoid supplemental megadoses (many times the daily recommended intakeof nutrients). Some can be toxic.

▶ *Vitamin B complex is the most important supplement; it can be taken at 100 mg of a full strength, yeast-free form.*

▶ *Vitamin C can be taken at a dose of up to 500 mg of a bioflavonoid complex twice daily.*

▶ *Two 30 mg zinc citrate tablets can be taken at night.*

▶ *Selenium is best taken in a combined formulation with vitamins A, C, and E.*

MAKING YOUR OWN JUICES

The raw juices of vegetables and fruits are excellent sources of vitamins, minerals, trace elements, and enzymes. For some people they are easier to take than whole foods and are generally very digestible. Juices are a good way to increase the level of antioxidant nutrients in the diet and may be used as an aperitif or a refreshing between-meal drink. Take a tumblerful at a time and sip the juice slowly. If you have a juicer, freshly squeezed juices are best, but canned or bottled juices are also good, as long as they are free of any additives or sweeteners (you can dilute pineapple juice half and half with water).

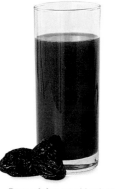

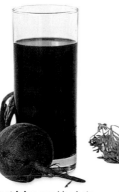

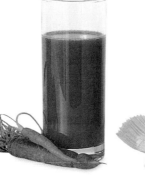

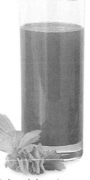

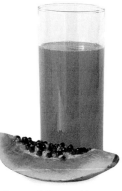

Prune juice provides beta carotene, potassium, and iron, excellent for boosting all-round health and vitality. It is also a useful laxative.

Beet juice provides beta carotene, folic acid, magnesium, potassium, calcium, and iron. It may improve blood disorders.

Carrot juice contains folic acid, beta carotene, vitamin C, potassium, magnesium, and phosphorus. Limit intake if you are diabetic.

Celery juice gives you potassium. It is good for lowering high blood pressure and rebalancing the adrenal function.

Papaya juice provides vitamin C, beta carotene, phosphorus, and potassium. It is also good for digestion problems.

INDEX

ACKNOWLEDGMENTS

Carroll & Brown Limited
would like to thank
Rachel Aris
Dr Edward Bach Centre
Bowtech
International Association for Colour
  Therapy
Michael Tse, Tse Qigong Centre

Photographic assistants
Lee McPherson
Colin Tatham
M.A. Hugo

Picture research
Richard Soar

Index
Jennifer Mussett

Photograph sources
   6 The Stock Market
   9 (Top) Science Photo Library
       (Bottom) US Library of
       Congress/Science Photo Library
  10 Oriental Museum, Durham
       University, UK/Bridgeman Art
       Library, London
  11 Science Photo Library
  12 Tony Stone Images
  21 Tony Stone Images
  26 (Top) Chris Priesti/Science
       Photo Library
       (Bottom) Wellcome Institute
       Library, London
  28 Hutchison Library
  34 (Left) E. Gueho/CNRI Science
       Photo Library
       (Right) Professor P.M. Motta
       et al/Science Photo Library
  36 The Image Bank
  40 The Image Bank
  43 (Left) Scott Camazine/Science
       Photo Library
       (Centre) The Stock Market
       (Top right) Sinclair Stammers/
       Science Photo Library

  (Right) Professor P.M. Motta
  et al/Science Photo Library
  (Bottom right) Claude
  Nuridsany & Marie Perennou/
  Science Photo Library
  44 (Top) Charron, Jerrican/Science
       Photo Library
       (Bottom) Corbis/Hulton
       Deutsche Collection
  45 Tibet Images
  46 Dr Edward Bach Centre
  46 The Image Bank
  48 Pictor International
  49 (Wood) Pictor International
       (Metal) Pictor International
  50 Science Museum/Science &
       Society Picture Library
  54 Kunsthistorisches Museum,
       Vienna/Bridgeman Art Library,
       London
  55 Tony Stone Images
  57 Tony Stone Images
  62 The Stock Market
  63 Tony Stone Images
  65 Eye of Science/Science Photo
       Library
  67 Elizabeth Whiting Associates/
       Andrew Kolesnikow
  68 Bowtech
  74 (Top) Smith Art Gallery and
       Museum, Stirling/Bridgeman Art
       Library, London
       (Bottom) Tony Stone Images
  76 Tony Stone Images
  78 Tony Stone Images
  95 (Left) Andrew Syred/Science
       Photo Library
       (Right) CNRI/Science Photo
       Library
 112 The Stock Market
 123 Michael Tse, Tse Qigong Centre
 126 Tony Stone Images
 128 The Stock Market
 132 The Stock Market
 136 Dr Gopal Murti/Science Photo
       Library
 149 NIBSC/Science Photo Library

Illustrators
Kim Dalziel
Rosamund Fowler
John Geary
Nicola Gregory
Halli Verinder
Anthea Whitworth
Paul Williams

Hair and make-up
Bettina Graham
Kim Menzies